Nursing Ethics

Ian E. Thompson
BA(Hons), PhD
Senior Educationalist, Scottish Health Education Group

Kath M. Melia
BNurs(Manc), SRN, HV, PhD
Lecturer, Department of Nursing Studies, University of Edinburgh

Kenneth M. Boyd
MA, BD, PhD
Scottish Director, Society for the Study of Medical Ethics

Churchill Livingstone 🏛

EDINBURGH LONDON MELBOURNE AND NEW YORK 1983

CHURCHILL LIVINGSTONE
Medical Division of Longman Group Limited

Distributed in the United States of America by Churchill Livingstone Inc., 1560 Broadway, New York, N.Y. 10036, and by associated companies, branches and representatives throughout the world.

First published 1983

ISBN 0 443 0230 8

British Library Cataloguing in Publication Data
Thompson, Ian E.
  Nursing ethics.
  I. Title.   II. Melia, Kath M.
  III. Boyd, Kenneth M.
  174'.2   RT85

Library of Congress Cataloging in Publication Data
Thompson, Ian E.
  Nursing ethics.
  1. Nursing ethics.   I. Melia, Kath M.
  II. Boyd, Kenneth M.   III. Title.   [DNLM:
  1. Ethics, Nursing.   WY T472n]
  RT85.T476   1983   174'.2   82–17696

Printed in Singapore by
The Print House (Pte) Ltd

Preface

Nursing ethics today is a subject of study in its own right. It can no longer be regarded simply as a branch of medical ethics or of ethics in general; nor can it be regarded simply as a matter of passing on hints and tips about manners and morals. In 1900, the American nurse Isabel Hampton Robb published a book with the same title as this one. In it, she stated that ethics 'teaches men the practice of duties of human life and the reasons for what they do and for what they should leave undone'.[1] Statements of that kind reflected the philosophical and popular confidence of the time that ethics was largely about doing your duty and that your duty was largely obvious. As far as nurses were concerned, it was summed up in the demand for 'implicit, unquestioning obedience',[2] and in the requirements of conventional respectability. Today, things are not so simple. The social and professional hierarchies within which modern nursing was established no longer seem part of an eternal order: nurses, while recognising a proper division of labour between themselves, medicine and the other health care occupations, no longer take the view that it is 'ours not to reason why'; and the study of ethics, in a plural, multicultural society, now supplies at least as many unsolvable moral dilemmas as clear ethical imperatives.

Changes of this kind, together with developments in medical science and technology, and evidence, this century, that even members of professions with high ideals can sometimes act unethically, has greatly increased professional and public interest in medical and nursing ethics. Interest in nursing ethics is now apparent in nursing conferences and the nursing press, as well as in the time increasingly being set aside for teaching of the subject in nursing curricula. All of this is an indication that in ethics as in other aspects of nursing practice, research and teaching, Florence Nightingale's dictum is again relevant.

What cruel mistakes are sometimes made by benevolent men and women in matters of business about which they can know nothing and think they know a great deal.[3]

In relation to nursing ethics, this advice points to the need for those with practical knowledge of nursing's real moral dilemmas now to engage in common study with those from other disciplines, including those with some skill in asking pertinent ethical questions and exploring their implications. If nursing ethics is to be taught or studied well, an interprofessional approach is necessary.

This book is largely the result of attempts to put this interprofessional approach into practice. The collaboration, in its authorship, of a philosopher, a nurse and a theologian arose out of their earlier co-operation in the work of the Edinburgh Medical Group and in nursing ethics teaching, particularly at Queen Margaret College, Edinburgh. The authors are particularly grateful to the staff and students of that college for stimulating their thinking and providing a great variety of helpful insights on the matters discussed in the book. They are also grateful to the group of nurses who met, when the book was first mooted, to explore the areas with which it might deal. In planning the book they were also fortunate in having the assistance of Dr Alison Tierney who, while not responsible for its defects and shortcomings, made many helpful suggestions about its form and content. Mrs Mary Law of Churchill Livingstone also has to be thanked for her patience and practical assistance.

The aims and methods of the book are outlined in the introduction which follows. Chapters 2 and 3 were written by Dr Melia, who is a Lecturer in Nursing Studies at the University of Edinburgh. Chapters 4 to 7 were written by Dr Thompson, who is a Senior Educationalist with the Scottish Health Education Group. The book was edited and the introduction written by Dr Boyd, who is Scottish Director of the Society for the Study of Medical Ethics. The authors hope that the book will be found useful not only for private study by nurses and others, but also in ethics seminars and courses of the kind out of which it arose.

1. Robb I H 1915 Nursing ethics. Cleveland, p 13
2. Robb I H 1915 Nursing ethics. Cleveland, p 57
3. Nightingale F 1980 Notes on nursing. In: Skeet M, Nightingale F Notes on Nursing. Churchill Livingstone, Edinburgh, p 111

Contents

1

Introduction

This book is about moral dilemmas in nursing and the ethics
of nursing care. How to deal with moral dilemmas, of course,
is not something anyone can learn from a book. It is a matter,
rather, of action and reflection on action, of making mistakes
and learning to live with the knowledge that we shall probably
make mistakes in the future. The most that this or any book
on the subject can do is to set out and criticise arguments for
and against the moral alternatives which face us, and to bring
to our attention ethical considerations which may not be
immediately obvious to us. A book of this kind, in other words,
is simply an extension of what happens when we discuss our
moral dilemmas and choices with other people. Thinking
about everyday moral dilemmas we almost inevitably begin by
seeing these from our own point of view: but if we listen atten-
tively to other people involved in the situation, or to an impartial friend, we often begin to see other sides to the question,
which, in turn, affect what we feel we ought to do. So in discussing moral dilemmas and choices generally, there usually
are more sides to the question and more kinds of relevant
moral arguments than we begin by recognising; and the aim
of a book of this kind is to identify and criticise some of these
different arguments. But having done that, the book has not

1

provided us with 'answers'. Learning to see our everyday moral choices through the eyes of others involved, or of an impartial adviser, may make us sympathetic or vulnerable to their points of view: but it does not make our choice for us. Similarly, when we study moral questions, we become aware of the variety of arguments for and against different alternatives, their strength and their weaknesses: but in the end this usually leaves us with more questions than answers, and the choice, in practice, remains our own. The advantage of studying the arguments, in other words, is much the same as the advantage of listening to other people: it expands our intellectual horizons in the hope that this will make us less self-centred and short sighted: but it does not make our choices for us, nor does it make choosing any easier.

With these general aims in view, the book is divided into two main sections. The second of these (Chapters 4 to 6) is about moral dilemmas concerned, respectively, with the nurse-patient relationship, with nursing groups of patients and with nurses and society. This section has been written by Dr Thompson from the point of view of moral philosophy, the academic discipline traditionally concerned with moral and ethical questions. A rather different approach has been attempted however in the first section (Chapters 2 and 3) by Dr Melia who, writing from the point of view of a nurse and a sociologist, sets the moral dilemmas and choices to be discussed in the context of the experience of becoming and being a nurse in the practically-oriented world of patient care and professional organisation. These two approaches, it is hoped, may help to indicate the breadth of the area with which ethics is concerned, as well as the depth of the issues it raises. In addition to these two main sections a final chapter by Dr Thompson examines some of the more theoretical philosophical questions involved in the preceding disccusion of moral dilemmas.

This first chapter also is concerned with broader issues. Nursing is only one area of life in which moral dilemmas and choices arise, and while it has many special features which we shall consider later, it also has much in common with the rest of our moral experience. By way of introduction therefore we shall begin by defining some terms and discussing what we mean by moral dilemmas and choices in everyday life, noting how these dilemmas and choices are related to the ways in which moral values may change over time.

Ethics and moral dilemmas

What, in the first place, do we mean by moral dilemmas and ethics? The words 'morals' and 'ethics' originally meant much the same thing, 'ethics' coming from Greek and 'morals' from its Latin equivalent. Both words referred to the general area of the rights and wrongs, in theory and practice, of human behaviour. In everyday usage 'moral' and 'ethical' can still be used more or less interchangeably, but a distinction has grown up between 'morals' and 'ethics'. 'Morals' (and also 'morality') now tends to refer to the standards of behaviour actually held or followed by individuals and groups, while 'ethics' refers to the science or study of morals—an activity, in the academic context, also often called moral philosophy. This distinction, however, is complicated by three popular ways of using the words. 'Ethics' can also be used to refer to the morals or morality of certain groups, such as the professions, and sometimes to the morals or morality of individuals: the implication behind this usage is that the morals or morality involved either have been codified or carefully worked out, or that they are in some sense high-minded. Associated with this idea of high-mindedness is the second popular use—that of both 'moral' and 'ethical' as terms of approval, the opposite of 'immoral' or 'unethical'. The third popular use seems to derive from the idea of ethics as the impartial study or science of morals: this use is seen when 'ethics' and 'ethical' seem to be preferred to 'morals', 'morality' and 'moral' because the latter are thought of as having some connection either with sex on the one hand or with religious dogmatism on the other; 'ethics' and 'ethical', by contrast, are thought of as involving something more cerebral and objective. However, there is no substantial reason for these associations of ideas, which are largely a matter of preference, only slightly if at all more justifiable than the habit of preferring 'ethical' to 'moral' apparently for no better reason than that it sounds more impressive.

Given this background of different usages then, what do we mean by a moral dilemma? A dilemma is a choice, of whatever kind, between two equally unsatisfactory alternatives. A moral choice is a choice involving our beliefs and feelings about what we fundamentally regard as good or right—our moral values or moral principles. Not all dilemmas are moral dilemmas—some dilemmas are the result of our not knowing the best means, in theory or practice, to an agreed end. Nor are all moral choices moral dilemmas, since in many cases we may well know what we ought to do, and the question is whether we will do it or not. What makes the choice a moral dilemma, rather, is the fact that it involves conflict between moral principles (what we believe we ought to do) or moral values (what we think of as, or feel to be, fundamentally good or important and thus value as something we should act upon). We feel, in other words, that certain moral values or principles would make us adopt one alternative, but also that others would make us adopt the other: but we cannot adopt both, and choosing the one means not only not choosing the other, but actually going against what the value or principle it represents would have us do.

Moral dilemmas in everyday life

Moral dilemmas of this kind arise from time to time in the lives of most people. A student has promised her classmates that she will write up their group project, which must be handed in to their tutor the next morning. Just after she has started to write, her closest friend telephones in great distress, wanting to see her right away because her fiancé has just broken off their engagement. A few days later the student is approached on a snowy street by an emaciated beggar who asks her for the price of a cup of tea. The student can easily afford to give him this, but the beggar clearly has alcohol on his breath and it is only ten o'clock in the morning. Later in the day the student meets her married sister who is worried about her fourteen year old daughter. The daughter has asked if she can go to the next town tomorrow with a girlfriend—to see a new film and come back on the late train. She says that the other girl's parents have agreed, but her mother is unable to contact them and is not sure that her daughter has told her the whole story.

Each of these experiences seems to involve a moral dilemma then, because a choice between conflicting moral values or principles seems to be involved in each case. The first experience involves on the one hand the moral principle that we should keep our promises: on this side of the dilemma there is also the moral value of being a good or dutiful student. On the other side there is the moral value of being a good friend: there is also the moral principle that we should help others in need. The conflict here is not between different things the student *wants* to do (her best friend or the group project may each in their own way be tiresome and the alternative a welcome excuse) but between different things which she feels she *ought* to do. Meeting the beggar, the student may want to give him the money—perhaps to get him out of the way, perhaps to make herself feel virtuous. But she may also feel that she ought not to, because it would not be in his interest to continue drinking himself to death. On the other hand, she may not want to give him the money—perhaps because she needs her only ten pence for her bus fare, perhaps because she is afraid the beggar may recognise her and pester her again. But she may also feel that she ought to give it, because as another adult the beggar has a right to decide what is best for himself —and, again, because one ought to help others in need. Her sister's dilemma too, involves the right of another person to decide what is best for themselves, but in this case is complicated because the other person is a child. If teenagers are to become responsible adults, parents have to learn to 'let go' and trust them to be responsible, even if this means letting them make their own mistakes. On the other hand some mistakes can have very serious consequences, and parents have a responsibility also to protect their children. If the mother values responsibility, that value will exert considerable moral pressure on both sides of her dilemma.

Moral dilemmas, information and communication

The examples we have discussed all seem to be of genuine unresolvable moral dilemmas. But certain facts might emerge which could call this in question. The student might have failed to read a notice from the tutor postponing the project deadline by a week. The beggar might have been at a crucial stage in voluntary psychiatric treatment for alcoholism. The other girl's parents might have agreed to her going to the cinema on the condition that one set of parents collected the two girls from there by car. In each case this vital information, if it had come to light, might well have resolved—or dissolved—the respective dilemma. In the case of the project this would be for obvious reasons. In that of the beggar, the student might be able to argue that because his psychiatric treatment was voluntary, her refusal of money was supporting his own prior decision about what was best for himself. As far as the girls were concerned, the information might allow the mother to negotiate an agreed compromise with her daughter about the degree of responsibility appropriate to the circumstances.

Possibilities of this kind illustrate the importance, when facing moral dilemmas in everyday life, of adequate information and good communication. Quite often, what appears to be a moral dilemma is the result of a breakdown in, or the absence of, relevant communication between different people. This is certainly true of some areas of inter-professional and professional-patient communication with which we shall be concerned later. (If a nurse does know what a doctor has told a dying patient, she may not be sure whether or not to give a truthful reply to the patient's question about what is happening to him. When the bed of a patient awaiting discharge is urgently needed for another patient, the nursing staff's failure to discover that a relative has just arrived at home to look after the first patient, and their consequent misconception that this patient has nowhere to go, could create an avoidable moral dilemma about priorities.) So sometimes, especially when the same kind of moral dilemma regularly occurs, rather than agonising over each dilemma, it may be worth asking whether institutional or personal networks of communication cannot be improved in some appropriate way, either by some organisational means or by those involved cultivating a greater degree of tact or ingenuity.

Moral dilemmas and moral choice

Improvements in communication clearly have a part to play in avoiding certain unnecessary moral dilemmas. On the other hand there may be a temptation, particularly among practically-minded people, to overestimate what can be achieved in this way. The student's dilemma, we might say, could have been avoided either if the college had had a better system of informing students, or if the student herself had cultivated the habit of checking notice boards more assiduously. Her sister's dilemma too might have been avoided had she worked harder, over a longer period of time, at communicating with her daughter. Even the dilemma involving the beggar might have been avoided had the student, on meeting him, talked with him in a way which would have elicited the vital information. In each of these suggestions, clearly, a way round the moral dilemma can be found, just as, often enough, it can be found in everyday life. On the other hand there are many situations in everyday life when no such way exists; and even when it does, and the acute moral dilemma can be avoided, the fact of moral choice, and moral conflict, remains.

To illustrate this fact, consider the examples again. Meeting the beggar, the student might have started to talk with him and he might just possibly have given her the vital information. But in thus delaying any decision about whether to give him the money until she had more information, the student was already acting in a way which—at that time, with the information she had—went against what, on one side of her dilemma, she felt she ought to do: it went against, that is, another adult's right to decide what was best for him. Her decision to seek more information in this case was thus not a morally neutral matter. She had in fact come down on one side of the dilemma and made a moral choice.

Prior moral choice might equally have been involved in any means by which the other two dilemmas could have been avoided. A better system of informing students might have been possible for the college only at the cost of choosing not to spend its limited resources on, say, library facilities or student amenities: a prior moral choice or even moral dilemma about priorities would have been involved here. Again, in cultivating the habit of checking notice boards more regularly the student might have been opting for this as part of a general style of living which gave greater priority to the demands of work than the demands of friendship. Here too moral choices would have been involved, as they would have been in her sister's decision to spend more time with her daughter—which might well have been at the expense of time spent on her own work or with her husband.

Even when ways exist of avoiding acute, painful or recurrent moral dilemmas then, this does not mean that moral choices are not being made. Such choices may have been made over a long period of time, as the characters of individuals, relationships or institutions were being formed. But the succession of small choices made every day by everyone, individually or collectively, is no less significant than the large choice which an acute or painful moral dilemma confronts us with. In this sense everything that we do to some purpose can be seen, in principle at least, as the result of some moral choice, made recently or long ago, by us as individuals or as part of present or past society.

What all this suggests then, is that moral dilemmas, which we may reasonably wish to avoid in everyday life, can nevertheless play a useful part in our understanding of the moral dimension of our experience. The point about moral dilemmas is that they demonstrate, more dramatically than other aspects of our experience do, the inescapability of moral choice in everyday life. A moral dilemma brings into sharper focus the moral values and principles which, even when they conflict with one another, matter to us because of our previous moral choices, many of which have been everyday and relatively unconsidered, but which cumulatively have gone to make up what we may call our moral character. Confronted by a moral dilemma, the fact that we recognise it as such challenges us also to recognise the strength of our conflicting values, and in making—or not making—a moral choice, to adopt, change or reinforce the nature of our moral character. In studying moral issues then, while it is reasonable enough to look—as we would in everyday life—for ways round or out of the dilemma, it is also useful to consider the dilemma on the assumption that there are no such ways, and to ask, if that is the case, which option we would choose and how we would defend our choice in the light of the values involved. When we have begun to do that, it might be added, we have begun to study ethics.

Shared and changing values

In what has been written so far, moral values have been discussed mainly in terms of the values of individuals. But values, of course, are something we share. This can be seen in the fact that morals and politics are not distinct activities, but part of a continuum. People, it is true, sometimes talk about politics as if it were only a matter of power for power's sake: but while power clearly is of importance to many politicians, politics is also concerned with ideals and purposes, and values play an important part in political as well as moral dilemmas. Some of the earliest moral philosophers, Aristotle for example, considered that the study of ethics was part of the study of politics; and clearly enough the purposes, values and principles which we have as individuals cannot be properly studied in isolation from those of the society and culture which have made us what we are.

The fact of shared, as well as individual, values is of obvious importance in considering the moral dilemmas and ethics of a profession such as nursing. Some of the ways in which becoming a nurse may create shared values among members of the profession, and also create conflicts with the individual's values, will be discussed in chapter two, and the relationship between moral rules and roles will be mentioned also in chapter seven. In the broader context of everyday moral choice, however, it may be worth asking here about how our shared values have been changing and what effect this may be having on our contemporary moral decision-making.

One of the major changes which seems to have taken place in our society during the last century is a shift from general public agreement about moral values to what we now call moral pluralism. Not everybody a hundred years ago, of course, agreed about what was morally right and wrong, nor today is society without consensus on some moral issues. But the variety of moral viewpoints which it is acceptable to express and possible to justify in public does seem to have become greater; and the fact that there are so many possible and defensible moral viewpoints may well be one reason why we are particularly aware today of moral conflicts and dilemmas. How we view this situation will depend on our moral presuppositions: some will see it as symptomatic of moral liberation, others of moral decay. The truth is probably, as usual, more complex, and because we are living through it, largely hidden from us. But on the basis of what has happened to societies in the past, one way of interpreting what is happening now may be by comparing it with the transition, in individuals, from childhood to adolescence.

An immediately obvious aspect of this comparison is the way in which many people today look back nostalgically to the lost moral certainties of the past. This backward nostalgic look is reminiscent of what, in retrospect, seems so attractive about childhood—its security and particularly the certainty of childhood ideas. Grandmother is a saint, father can do anything, our family's ways are the best ways, the others are rather odd. The pain, but also the excitement, of adolescence lies in discovering that things are really much more complicated and often not what they seemed. Grandmother can be an emotional tyrant, father has not conquered the world, other families' ways and moral standards may be as good as, if not better than, ours. The change experienced in adolescence, in other words, is from a world in which things are morally black and white to one in which we discover an infinite variety of moral shades of grey. In this situation we are faced with two major temptations. One is to deny that the shades of grey exist, possibly by adopting a new black and white morality supplied by some moral, religious or political dogmatic ideology: the dangers in this are those of moral myopia about the complexity of real-life decision-making and moral insensitivity towards those with different convictions. The other temptation is to accept the infinite variety of moral shades of grey and to say that they are all the same, it is all relative, it does not matter what you do: the dangers here are those of moral indifference and moral indecisiveness.

One way of understanding what has been happening to morality in our society then is to compare it with this transition from the moral certainties of childhood to the uncertainties, temptations and dangers of adolescence. Similar changes have taken place in the past, when individuals or societies have experienced the transition from tribal or village life to the life of large cosmopolitan cities. In the tribe or village, morality was a matter of shared fixed conventions which gave people considerable security—but at the price, often, of hypocrisy, guilt and even open cruelty towards those who deviated from the moral norm. The shift to city life, where people from different origins with different moral views lived together, made it difficult to maintain the old black and white certainties, revealed the moral shades of grey and exposed individuals and society to the adolescent's temptations of moral dogmatism and moral relativism. In our time, something of the same kind seems to have been happening to society generally through the growth of travel, communication, the media and education. These developments have made more people than ever before aware of the variety of moral viewpoints which it is possible to hold, and consequently of the difficulty, in the face of this, of maintaining that any one traditional moral viewpoint is right or the best.

Against this background, one particular value which has fallen in public esteem is that of paternalism and the principle that 'father knows best'. This shift is associated with greater respect for the value of self-determination and the idea of human rights—especially the rights of women and of minorities. Involved in this change also is an emphasis on the individual which favours such values as self-expression rather than self-sacrifice, tolerance rather than conformity, and flexibility rather than strict obedience to moral rules. Changes of this kind seem to be reflected today in changing attitudes within nursing, traditionally a female, obedient, self-sacrificing and sometimes rigid profession. These changing attitudes focus on questions about the authority of the traditionally male profession of medicine, the separate identity of nursing as a profession in its own right and the need for more flexible ways of providing care. Changing values also seem to be reflected in contemporary concern for such things as the patient's right to know and the right to self-determination in health care.

This account of changing attitudes and moral values in our society is suggested here merely as one impression of what has been happening; and it can be immediately conceded that the changes suggested are far from universal. That such changes are far from universal is, in fact, part of the point we are making here, since a major difficulty in moral decision-making today lies in the unpredictability of the values held by other people. Frequently, in other words, it is not possible to rely in moral dilemmas and choices on an appeal to values which, in the past, might have been expected to command general support. In nursing, for example, there is still considerable reluctance to go on strike, but this reluctance cannot be relied upon as much as in the past; and it is likely to be defended only in some cases by an appeal to the traditional values of duty and obedience: in other cases the defence is more likely to be in terms of the value of care or concern for patients, or even of the profession's self-interest where striking is thought to be counter-productive.

As this example suggests, the variety of moral values which different people hold today is a matter of practical concern as well as of theoretical interest. Conflict between moral values exists not only on either side of the moral dilemmas confronted by individuals, but also within society and between different societies. The great divisions in today's world are not only about material issues of power, wealth and poverty, but also about which moral values should have priority in the ordering of society: should liberty be put first, as in Western societies, or equality as in Socialist, or the law of God as in resurgent Islam? Moral conflicts of this kind, clearly, can spill over into social, economic and even physical conflict within societies as well as between them; and while political bargaining can play some part in the attempt to reconcile different interests, the purposes, ideals and values which move individuals and societies to action must also be taken into account if the harmful consequences of conflict are to be avoided.

In seeking to avoid these harmful consequences, it is important to remember that moral conflict in itself is not bad. Indeed it is only through moral conflict that society can resist the temptations of moral dogmatism and moral relativism and thus remain responsive to the variety of moral values which makes life fully human. But to resist these temptations and at the same time to avoid the harmful consequences of conflict is not easy, and perhaps not even possible, unless individuals and societies have some way of communicating with one another which helps each to understand the importance of the other's moral values without thereby diminishing the the importance of their own. In human life, clearly, there are many ways of establishing such communication, ranging from marriage to international diplomacy. But one useful way, we would suggest in the present context, is through the kind of reasoned public debate about moral issues which we undertake in the study of ethics. Such debate provides a framework within which people can communicate with one another about the values and principles which move them to action; a framework within which they can give one another reasons why they believe these values and principles to be important, can offer and listen to reasonable criticism and can, on occasion, find ways of establishing public consensus about the rights and wrongs of particular conflicts. In an area such as health care, at a time when recourse is increasingly been made to the courts and to political bargaining, ethics would seem to have a particularly useful contribution to make.

To say this, of course, is not to suggest that we all need to become philosophers any more than we are all able to be saints. Nor is it to suggest that someone who has mastered the technical language of ethics is necessarily thereby a better person or even someone better able to resolve moral difficulties in practice—the opposite indeeed is often the case. But it does suggest that to make ourselves vulnerable to, and critical of, the ethical arguments and moral sentiments of others is to respond in a more creative and constructive way to the moral complexity and conflicts of our time than by retreating either into moral dogmatism or into moral relativism. Vulnerability, indeed, is probably the key word here. Moral dogmatism and moral relativism are each in their own ways attempts to be invulnerable to moral conflict, by pretending either that we have no doubts, or that none of it matters. But the point which we have been trying to make in this introductory chapter and which, we hope, will be apparent in the chapters which follow, is that moral conflict does matter and that, in practice, we can rarely be entirely sure that our actions have always been right or for the best. This is particularly true of the field of health care, where professionals are frequently required to act quickly and decisively in matters affecting the vital interests of patients. To ask such professionals also to be vulnerable to such knowledge, and thus to the pain and guilt it may involve, is no doubt hard. But it is only in accepting such vulnerability, perhaps, that any of us escapes from moral adolescence into precarious adulthood.

2

Becoming and being a nurse

The decision to become a nurse may well be made in much the same way as the decision to become anything else—an architect, say, or a secretary or a market gardener. In the case of nursing, however, the word 'become' is more apt than it is for many other occupations. Becoming a nurse is not simply a matter of learning particular skills and adopting forms of behaviour appropriate to particular contexts. It is also a matter of coming to know the values of a profession in a way which can profoundly influence the thinking, personality and life-style of the individual concerned.

The process of becoming a nurse, and the conflicts it involves, are important aspects of the ethics of nursing care, concerned as this is not only with isolated moral dilemmas but also with character, roles and relationships. In this chapter, therefore, we shall discuss some relevant aspects of what it means to become and be a nurse. We shall consider first the difference between professional and lay nursing, together with some of the moral conflicts which this raises for the learner. Moral conflict, however, does not cease, although its nature may change, when the student gains her professional qualifications. In the later part of the chapter therefore we shall discuss some of the moral conflicts which arise in the context of the nurse's relationship with patients. Then, in the next chapter, we shall turn to some moral issues of a different kind which arise in the sphere of the nurse's relationship with other professionals.

Nursing, lay and professional

Those entering the nursing profession normally bring with them a lay conception of nursing and hence often do not realise that their chosen work will involve difficult decisions which may call into question their own personal convictions and values. Today, of course, the lay conception of nursing involves some appreciation of the difficulties and conflicts faced by health professionals. Discussion in newspapers and on television has made the general public very aware of ethical issues in health care. Nevertheless, it is probably true to say that nurses are not generally thought to have responsibilities or conflicts of such magnitude as those encountered by doctors. Doctors are highly specialised and skilled, and in the popular view they are often seen as dealing daily with 'life and death' matters. The lay view of nursing, by contrast, is probably less dramatic. Nursing, moreover, is something which lay people themselves do: it is, after all, carried out by members of the family at home and by untrained, as well as trained, personnel in hospitals. The lay view of nursing, in other words, may make it difficult for the newcomer to the profession to appreciate the responsibilities and complexities and hence the moral conflicts which she will have to encounter.

In order to appreciate these responsibilities, complexities and conflicts here, it is necessary to look a little further at the similarities and differences between lay and professional nursing. Looking after a sick relative at home involves doing things for the patient which he cannot do for himself, preventing the patient from undertaking any activity which will impede his recovery and administering any treatment or medication which has been prescribed. Leaving aside some of the technicalities of modern hospital care, and allowing professionals a greater degree of relevant information and resources, these are essentially the same activities which a qualified nurse would undertake either in the home or in hospital. In terms of what nursing involves at a practical level therefore, it is difficult to establish how the care given by a lay person differs from that provided by nurses. Nevertheless the two do differ, in at least three fundamental ways. First, nurses undertake their work not on the basis solely of duty, altruism or necessity, but on a contractual basis. Professional nurses look after patients in return for payment and, in the case of trainee nurses, to gain their professional qualifications. Second, nurses and patients are not normally personally involved in each other's lives in any sphere other than the nurse-patient relationship. Lay nursing, by contrast, usually takes place within the context of a family or of friendship, thus involving a different kind of carer-patient relationship. Third, the nurse and patient in the professional setting may well come from different backgrounds and thus not share the same outlook, culture, values and expectations.

The transition from lay to professional

Factors of this kind, which distinguish professional from lay nursing, may help to point to some of the problems encountered in the transition from lay to professional role. During the transition, or socialisation process, the learner discovers and adopts the professional approach to nursing in terms both of practical skills and of attitudes and values. The latter may cause particular problems. In the context of lay nursing, differences in values may raise difficulties, either across generations or between individuals. But such difficulties arise against the background of a lifetime of family differences and agreed ways of negotiating them. The needs of the individual, rather than the demands of a large organisation, moreover, are the pivot of decision-making. In professional nursing, by contrast, there exist not only institutional pressures but also the need for coexistence between the values of an individual and of a profession. The risk of conflict between these personal and professional values is at its height during the early years of training, when the new recruit has not yet been socialised to the extent of having adopted for herself the values of the profession.

The risk of such conflict is particularly acute in nursing because, while socialisation may be incomplete, the transition at a functional level has to happen very quickly. The learner spends a short time at the college of nursing absorbing some of the basic tenets of nursing care, and she has a chance to visit the hospital wards to see these in practice. But then one day the student finds herself standing in a ward, a patient calls 'Nurse': and he means her. At this functional level then, the student abandons her lay status almost overnight. What then of the deeper adjustments she must make? When does she feel like a nurse?

It is in such experiences of being and yet still becoming a nurse that the learner meets her first conflicts. She has to confront on the one hand her own personal feelings and reactions to the situations in which she finds herself, and on the other the values and attitudes of the professional group which she has joined. For example:

A learner is being shown around her new ward by the staff nurse. It is a geriatric ward, and clearly a busy one. She has been told that after a 'quick' tour she is to work with a third year student and that by such an arrangement they should 'get straight by lunchtime'. Half way down the ward there is a lady in her eighties, sitting by her bed. As they approach she asks the learner for the time and what is for lunch, and whilst asking she secures a firm grip of her uniform skirt. The staff nurse announces loudly that Mrs Black is always asking the same questions because she is demented and has a grossly impaired memory. She gives the newcomer no indication as to how she is to extricate herself from the situation whilst conveying very clearly the message that she is to follow her down to the dayroom to complete her tour of the ward.

In this situation the personal moral code of the learner might very well dictate that she stay and talk with the patient. At this level it matters little whether the patient is demented or not: she is another human being who has started a conversation with her. All the learner's past experience of life tells her to provide an answer and to conduct the conversation as she might any other. However, within the context of nursing, this old lady's request for information has been re-interpreted as the product of her dementia and as such can and should legitimately be ignored so that the 'real' work of nurses might progress.

Socialisation and sensitivity

Such a situation demonstrates the initial sensitivity which new-comers to the nursing profession possess while at the same time indicating how, once the professional approach to the work is adopted, this initial sensitivity becomes threatened. This desensitising process is to a large extent synonymous with the socialisation process. Much of the difficulty involved in 'becoming' a nurse is bound up with feelings of inadequacy and an inability to cope with the reactions which the intro-duction to nursing provokes in an individual. The newcomer has no stock of responses to these new encounters, such as with patients in pain, dependent sick adults, young cancer vic-tims, the products of road traffic accidents. Her past experi-ence, her values and her own moral convictions might yield a set of emotional responses to these new encounters, but they do not provide any prescription for action or reaction. The new recruits thus soon adopt the ways of nursing which they see around them. This can be said to be due, in part, to their lack of alternatives and in part to the efficiency of the socialisation process.

One of the consequences of an efficient socialisation pro-cess is the appearance of well-ordered professional behaviour, with everyone assuming an air of confidence and security in the knowledge that their behaviour is in line with the 'profes-sional way'. This makes life even more difficult for the new-comers as they tend to feel that everyone is coping except themselves. Learners might well think that they are the only ones to feel shocked by some of the sights they meet, for example, the soon to be taken-for-granted sight of so much nakedness, the lack of privacy and a seemingly matter-of-fact approach to human suffering. These feelings of shock, revul-sion, or simply of inadequacy, are further evidence of the naivety and sensitivity of the new recruits to nursing. Yet the concurrent suggestion, often made by learners them-selves, that they should not register any such feelings, reveals the fact that already they have some notion of the profession-al attitude towards such feelings. It is more probably these early observations which make the trainee nurse aware that she is weighing up nursing against her own standards. The first sighting of a surgical wound, a colostomy, an amputee or a demented patient, and above all the experience of caring for dying patients, can profoundly shock the recently-arrived learner. It is in terms of such encounters that the junior nurse confronts her personal feelings and values with the professional values of nursing.

The speed with which the new recruits adopt the prevailing mode of nursing has both advantages and disadvantages. On the positive side it affords the learner some fairly immediate way of coming to terms with what she sees, and of finding a way of functioning. By looking around her she sees what others do, others who are seemingly coping and not distressed by what they see, and follows suit. The disadvantage in the newcomer so readily adopting the 'professional' approach to nursing is, as has already been suggested, that she puts at risk her initial sensitivity, where personal moral values dominated. An example might be the way in which the toilet needs of patients on a geriatric ward are met. A trainee nurse might well be initially offended by the idea of several old ladies being supplied with commodes *en masse* and with little privacy. As the weeks go by, however, she will become accustomed to such practices and even if she does not come fully to accept them she is less likely to see the offensive side of the situation and to move towards an appreciation of the justifications upon which this 'professional' approach to the patient care rests.

Because the newcomer is at a loss as to how to behave when faced with patients, she will often feel silly and incompetent. Her major concern might well be to find some way of coping and meeting the expectations of the trained staff. In so doing, the learner can be well aware that she is compromising her own value system in the way that she feels she must behave towards patients. For example, hospital mealtimes are often rushed affairs, where the main nursing objective might well appear to a newcomer to be to serve meals and collect in plates, empty or otherwise, in the shortest space of time. A learner, given the task of feeding a reluctant patient, is often placed in a situation where she feels obliged to hurry the patient in order to satisfy the expectations of the staff. At the same time, she feels a natural response of sympathy for the patient and, following her own personal instincts, might be disinclined to hurry him or, if he is very reluctant, even to feed him. Again, there is a conflict between the preferred individual behaviour of the learner and that of the professional nurse.

The organisation of nursing

The distinction between lay and professional approaches to nursing can be elaborated in terms of the organisation of nursing in order to provide some further understanding of the conflicts which the professional style of nursing presents. Lay nursing is essentially organised upon an individual basis—one patient with one or more carers—who, importantly, know each other. The way in which the nursing is carried out is thus constrained, for the most part, only by the needs of this small group of people. The lay activity of nursing is able to follow a pattern based on a set of values normally worked out over a long period of time. Professional nursing, on the other hand, is usually carried out on a larger scale and involves people who do not know each other. Professional nursing activity is thus organisationally oriented and operates along the lines of routine approaches to care. Routines are less capable of accommodating individuals with regard to their individuality in terms of their needs and value systems. This lack of emphasis upon the individual is true for both patients and nurses. It should perhaps be noted that the college of nursing teaches its recruits nursing in the individual style. The patient is the central focus and the learners are taught to plan care along individualised lines according to individual needs. This 'lay'-type approach denies the reality of the routinised 'professional' approach to nursing which is to be found on many wards.

Roles and individuals

Professional nursing within an organisation relies upon the notion of role rather than individual. That is to say there are several roles, for example nurse, patient, relative, doctor and so forth, into which individuals are placed. Their expected behaviour within the organisation is determined by the role and not the person. This arrangement means that a certain uniformity is introduced into the system, for along with each role goes a set of expectations, responsibilities and privileges.

In practical terms, this means that certain forms of behaviour can be expected of the incumbents of different roles: the nurse is expected to care for patients in such a way as the whole body of professional nurses would recognise and deem fit. Similarly a patient, whoever he is, is expected to follow the dictates of his carers, to be grateful for his care and do his best to comply with his treatment. In this way an organisation such as a hospital can function without every individual having to start from first principles with everyone he meets. The rules of behaviour, in other words, are laid down and adherence to role expectations by individuals is the key to the success of such an organisation.

There remains, however, one problem. That individuals adopt roles is only one side of the coin: for they also retain their individuality. The individual who adopts the role of nurse takes on the legal and moral obligations of nursing as defined by statute and the profession. But at the same time she does not relinquish her individual character with its personal morality, beliefs and values. It is the very fact of the co-existence of personal values and professional values which presents many practical and ethical problems for nurses.

Routine and compromise

The mainstay of the professional approach to nursing is routine. Nursing care can be reduced to a set of routines which are designed to meet the needs of a group of patients. Patients have individual needs, but in their role of 'patient' they can be added to other patients and their overall needs provided along organised professional nursing lines rather than lay individual lines. In this way the nursing care of a group of patients can be conceived of as a workload to be got through. One of the most efficient ways in which to do this is to divide the care up into a series of tasks and share them, and incidentally the patients, among the nurses. This practice faces the learner with a further kind of conflict—to decide whether she should hold on to the principles of 'good' nursing which she has been taught and proceed along the individualised care lines put forward by the college, or simply to join the routine care which is being practised. In the event she has little choice, since being a junior nurse she will invariably do as she is told. However, this does not remove the conflict, since the learner has the added problem of living with her conscience if she feels she has compromised her own judgement and acted against the interests of the patients.

Unfortunately, at this early stage, whilst the student is still able to see what goes on in nursing with new eyes, she is also preoccupied with becoming a nurse, that is with behaving as other nurses do. By the time the recruit has become accustomed to the work, is less frightened and perplexed by the realities of nursing, she has probably also lost some of that initial innocence. To return again to an earlier example, new nurses are often struck by the dehumanising aspects of hospital care. Patients appear to have very little control over their life in hospital, there is greatly reduced privacy and intimate procedures and issues are often treated seemingly lightly. The new nurse's perspective on all of this is in some ways closer to the lay perspective of the patient than it is to that of the professional nurse. She is still in the process of transition from the lay to the professional perspective and thus can empathise with the patient. At this early stage, however, she is in no real position to influence the style of care given. By the time she does reach a stage when she feels that she might exert her own views and carry out her nursing according to her own judgements, there is a danger that the sights which initially offended her and provoked a desire to respond in a way which was not congruent with professional values, are now commonplace. This need not necessarily mean that the learner has lost all touch with her lay approach to nursing and its attendant personal values. But it may mean that the actual consideration of the ethical implications of seemingly straightforward nursing work must now be a conscious positive activity, rather than a spontaneous reaction.

The process of 'becoming' a nurse, it might be added here, is in some ways similar to that of becoming a patient. The loss of a certain amount of identity, taking on a generalised role and behaving accordingly, are experiences common to nurse and patient. The student has a uniform, the patient nightwear; decisions about day-to-day living have been taken from the person and placed in the hands of the organisation, for example meal times, off-duty for the nurse, waking and sleeping times for the patient. New nurses often feel that they are in a rather rigid hierarchy which relies upon rank and punitive measures rather than rationality and reason. Their freedom to act and question what they see is sometimes restricted. This leaves many of the conflicts of personal and professional values unresolved.

The process of 'becoming' a nurse then is one which requires the recruit to adopt an approach to nursing which is consistent with that adopted by the profession as a whole. The socialisation process is an efficient one, since few lay people have the resources to cope with the demands of nursing as an individual, and hence newcomers opt for the security which goes with adopting the profession's values. The safety in numbers dictum only goes so far, however, as each individual nurse has still to cope with any discontinuities which may exist between her personal values and those of the profession. Such discontinuities do not cease with qualification. Up to this point we have studied two kinds of moral questions facing the learner. How can personal and professional values be reconciled? And how can the individual nurse practise 'good' nursing in the face of accepted compromise? Having become a nurse, the individual finds that these questions, although sometimes now easier to avoid, do not go away.

Relationships and feelings

One area in which such questions continue to arise is that of building up relationships with patients. From their earliest days in college, nurses have been made aware of the importance of building up a relationship between themselves and patients. If patients are to gain the maximum benefit from nursing care, they must trust the nurse who gives it. Part of the nurse's work, she is taught, is to educate the patient; and his education will be most effective when the nurse can tailor it to the individual's needs within a good nurse-patient relationship. The same advice is sometimes given in a different way by saying that patients must be considered as persons. But how does this total patient care approach work out in practice? It suggests that the nurse should become intimately acquainted with a number of patients. But these patients will be people towards whom the nurse is likely to have the normal range of human feelings. And alongside the advice to build relationships with patients as people, the nurse will also constantly hear the advice not to 'become involved'.

In formal terms, the advice to treat patients as persons involves respect for the individual patient's rights as well as for what the nurse or the health care system may consider to be his interests. But in terms of the nurse's feelings about actual people, there clearly may be difficulties and conflicts. The nurse may well feel much more empathy with, say, a young leukaemic patient of her own age than with an elderly demented patient at the end of his life—or for whatever personal reasons it may be the other way round. In the nurse's everyday life outside her sphere of work, the fact that there are some people she takes to, some she dislikes, and many about whom she has no very strong feelings, is something she may take for granted on the assumption that it takes all sorts to make a world. But when much the same mixture of people arrive as patients, the demands of building up a relationship and treating patients as persons make things much more difficult. The nurse, clearly, cannot be forced to like people to whom she may feel an aversion, any more than the patient with similar feelings towards the nurse can be forced to like her. Under these circumstances the nurse may adopt the Hippocratic maxim 'first, do not harm' to ensure that an instinctive dislike is not reflected in her overt attitudes. She may also be grateful for the positive feelings—including generalised sexual attraction—which make it easier to treat certain patients as persons. But in the end, the nurse will still remain prey to a range of human feelings towards other people whose potential for harm as well as good is never entirely suppressed by professional socialisation.

The fact that nurses have human feelings towards patients and that these feelings have a potential for harm as well as good clearly lies behind the advice not to 'become involved'. How far each nurse heeds this advice, and how far she finds it incompatible with building relationships with patients as persons, must ultimately be a matter for her own judgement. But her judgement is not formed in isolation and there are factors in the nurse's interactions with her seniors, her peers and patients which may exert an unrecognised influence on her. One such factor is the practice of 'labelling' patients.

Labelling patients

The notion of labelling comes from the sociology of deviance and has to do with our attitudes to people with attributes which we do not consider normal. Nurses, for example, may refer to patients as 'difficult' or 'unco-operative' or to their behaviour in terms of 'he won't help himself', 'just trying it on', 'doesn't want to get well' and so forth. In this way behaviour exhibited by the patient, which makes the nurse's work more difficult, is deemed to be deviant. By implication, this makes the nurse the innocent party in any encounter—a position which she strengthens by drawing upon the support of her colleagues in the use of the label. For example:

A patient who is used to working shifts does not like to settle early to sleep and prefers either to watch late-night television or to read. The nurse whose job is to follow hospital policy and turn her ward lights out by 10.30 p.m., finds this patient difficult to cope with. Because he feels strongly about staying up, the patient makes a great fuss each night and wins his fight to watch the late television film. The nurses when handing over shifts report that he is 'being awkward' again. In the patient's terms, this simply means going to bed at his usual time.

When nurses use this technique of labelling, then, it serves to legitimise the feelings that individual nurses may have towards a patient. The nurse can then think in terms which make, say, her own impatience with a patient seem not her own fault. In the case, for example, of a patient who is making very slow progress from a stroke, the nurses may have applied the label of 'doesn't try', which in turn shields the nurse who tries to get the patient dressed in the morning from her own feelings of frustration or even anger. When labelling is used in large institutions such as hospitals, moreover, the labelled behaviour can take on the character of a stereotype. The term 'awkward patient', for example, is then more than simply a description of one individual. It conjures up for the nurse a whole set of forms of behaviour expected from any patient thus labelled. To some extent, of course, such labelling and stereotyping is an inevitable part of social interaction. But the patient's vulnerability and dependence on the nursing staff mean that it has more far-reaching effects in his case than in everyday life. It is particulary important therefore that the nurse should be aware of what she is doing in applying or agreeing to a label. Is the label really accurate? Or is it simply a way of defending or excusing herself at the patient's expense?

Not all labels, of course, are of the kind described so far. A patient might be labelled as 'dependent', 'a child', 'dying' or 'mentally retarded', and labels of this kind can have some functional significance. They are not, of course, necessarily labels which the patient himself would agree with: and again, even category labels of this kind can be used in ways which are less in the interests of the patient than in that of the professional's own self-justification. There are however a number of category labels whose use has achieved a degree of consensus among health carers, and in discussing the moral questions we are concerned with further, it may be useful to look at one or two of these in greater detail.

Difficult and unpopular patients

Patients can be labelled as 'difficult' for a variety of reasons. A demanding elderly patient, a private patient who treats nursing staff as paid servants or a non-compliant patient all tend to attract this description. The old lady who rings her bell every time the nurse leaves the room is clearly as entitled to the services of the nurse as the lady in the next room who hardly ever asks for anything. Nevertheless the nurse is likely to feel annoyed with the old lady who 'wastes' her time and may often be tempted to use minor sanctions against her, or to resort to delaying tactics. Any attempt to justify this understandable kind of response, however, must overcome the objection that the nurse, being the stronger party in the relationship, has a greater responsibility to act in a just or fair way towards the weaker. Treating patients as people, in other words, involves respecting their rights—even when they seem to abuse them.

The nurse's problem in handling her own feelings is more complicated however when conflicting demands arise. The nurse may feel antagonistic to an alcoholic or 'overdose' patient, who seems to have brought his troubles upon himself.

But when a young girl, say, who has taken an overdose is brought in to a casualty department—to be followed within minutes by the victims of a serious road accident—the nurses who are left to look after the girl may well feel that they could be better employed working with the more 'deserving' accident victims. Similar problems may arise among nurses working in gynaecological words, where those having terminations may be nursed alongside infertile women who desperately want children. In situations of this kind, judgemental labelling may be a strong temptation for those whose personal moral values create antagonism. Unpopular patients consequently may be at some risk of having their psychological, if not physical needs undervalued. Here again any tendency in this direction has to be met by the demands of justice on the nurse.

Psychiatric labelling

In considering the demands of justice, one aspect of the nurse's stronger position is her special knowledge. In relation to labelling, this may involve more than simply giving a patient 'a bad name' in terms, such as 'difficult', 'rude' or 'demanding', which might be used by anyone. The nurse, because of her special knowledge, is in a position to misuse, as well as use, legitimate clinical labels. Typical examples of this come from the field of psychiatry. A patient who is unsettled in his hospital surroundings may well display strange behaviour: he may be rather aggressive towards people, or emotionally very labile or he may refuse to talk to anyone. The words which nurses use to describe this behaviour to each other may very easily take on the apparently objective overtones of a clinical diagnosis. For example:

> If a patient is rather low in spirits one evening because her husband is away on business and cannot visit her for a few days, the nurse might write in the Kardex 'fairly low tonight'. At the morning report she may say that the patient is still 'rather down'. By lunchtime the report is passed on that the patient is 'a bit depressed'. The label 'depressed' then finds its way into the Kardex. The changeover of staff on the next day means that the original user of 'low' is no longer on duty, so that the reason—the husband's absence—gets lost and

the depression label gains momentum to the extent that the houseman is asked to prescribe something for the patient.

The dangers of using clinical labels which have quite specific meanings in psychiatry in this way are clear. Labelling of this kind is in the best interests neither of the patient nor of nursing. If nurses are prepared to describe individual patients in derogatory or misleading terms, this is likely to affect the kind of care which they give. It also seems clear, from the literature on deviance, that persons are often labelled as deviant simply because they do not confrom to the norm. But how do nurses decide what should be classed as normal? Even if a consensus about normality can be arrived at by nurses, what right does one group have to decide that the behaviour of another is not acceptable and thus refuse to tolerate it?

Minority Groups

Questions of this kind may arise in the case of minority religious or ethnic groups which have values or cultural practices differing from the majority of the population. The hospital care of patients from such groups may well infringe their rights as individuals. In some cases, such as that of Jehovah's Witnesses requiring blood transfusions, the moral issues can be very complex. An example is discussed in Chapter 4. But other cases may be resolvable if the nurses involved are reasonably sensitive and flexible. For example:

A young nurse was in charge of a medical ward on night duty when a Jewish patient died. The nursing officer had warned her that she should move the patient from the ward before the relatives arrived, since once they started to mourn no-one would be allowed to touch the body. But in fact it was difficult to interfere in any way because the relatives had arrived and put candles round the bed some time before the patient died. The patient was moved into a side ward before he died—propped up on pillows and surrounded by his family. Later, the nurse was reprimanded for not laying the body down flat, in the normal way. But the nurse had realised that the Jewish faith insisted that no Gentile touch the patient and had decided to abide by their rules.

This nurse's problem might of course have been solved in a practical way by ensuring that the family was on hand to carry out the funeral arrangements as they saw fit. The example does however illustrate problems which can and do arise when hospital policy or personnel are too rigid to accommodate the wishes of a minority group. The organisational machine—or mind—which insists that certain rules must be followed, can sometimes make it very difficult for a single nurse to do what she thinks is right for the patient. In the example given, for instance, a more junior nurse might have felt less secure in her position and, despite knowing about the Jewish faith, might have laid the patient flat.

In circumstances of this kind, of course, as many more experienced nurses might well point out, the potential for flexibility within nursing and the individual nurse's capacity to work around the rules of the organisation may provide one way of resolving difficulties in protecting patient's rights. If, that is, a nurse knows why the hospital or health authority requires certain forms of behaviour from its nurses, she might then be in a position to 'bend the rules'. For example, part of the routine surgical admission of patients includes the patient having a bath. Clearly, in some cases, depending on the patient's circumstances, this may be desirable if not indeed necessary. On the other hand, to insist that every patient has a bath on admission not only may be unnecessary, but could give offence. It is not a particularly good way in which to 'build the relationship' either. Thus, once the nurse understands the reason for this traditional practice—namely, that at one time the general standard of hygiene was poor—she is in a position to attempt to waive the rules when appropriate. In justifying her desired action to her seniors she can invoke the reasoning behind the practice and demonstrate that as an inflexible rule it is not only redundant but possibly counterproductive in terms of human relations. Such conduct on the part of a junior nurse however may well require some courage: and in nursing, as in life generally, there is never any ultimate guarantee that other people will accept what to us is simply listening to reason.

In this chapter then we have explored some of the moral conflicts involved in becoming and being a nurse. We have considered the conflicts between personal values and routine practice in the transition from lay to professional status and the potential loss of sensitivity through too-successful socialisation. We have looked also at the conflict between treating patients as people and 'not becoming involved', and discussed the dangers of labelling. These are, of course, only some of the moral issues and conflicts involved in patient-care aspects of becoming and being a nurse. But perhaps they give some indication of the variety of moral choices which nurses have to make on a day-to-day basis not only during their training but throughout their professional careers. To conclude this chapter something further should be said about one of the most difficult aspects of nursing care, and one which many nurses would concede they have never entirely come to terms with, the experience of caring for dying patients.

The nurse and dying patients

Lay and professional nursing of dying patients are obviously different experiences, not least by virtue of the ties of family or friendship which normally bind the dying to their lay carers. Even when death is a relief, the experiences of a lifetime's closeness, together with the memories of happiness and hurt, have to be worked through; and especially when the inevitability of death is recognised, the working through may begin before death itself takes place. Professional nursing, by contrast, normally has no such fund of experiences to work upon. This does not mean however that the professional nurse is not vulnerable to the hopes, fears and present experiences of the dying individual. The experience of being in hospital is one which can allow people to speak more freely than normally about themselves; and the relationship between nurse and patient, however temporary, can be very important to the patient, not least because of his dependence on the nursing staff. How important the relationship is to the nurse will depend, of course, on how far she heeds the advice not to become involved. Nurses, clearly, cannot build up close relationships with all of their patients, even when nursing is undertaken on a patient-centred rather than task-oriented basis. But inevitably, for a great variety of reasons—perhaps because the patient reminds the nurse of her father, perhaps because the patient chose this nurse to confide her domestic troubles to—some patients will be of particular importance to some nurses, and their encounter with one another, however brief, will leave 'unfinished business' which the nurse must work through in her own emotions.

As a professional, of course, the nurse will feel it important that her own emotional demands do not get in the way of skilled caring. This may be particularly difficult if the death of such a patient occurs at a time when the nurse herself is feeling low for reasons rooted in her domestic or personal life, or through factors such as menstruation whose existence is not always recognised by organisational demands. Under these circumstances, if the patient's death occurs at a particularly busy time, the pressure of other work may either give the nurse the strength to postpone working through her emotions until she can find some time on her own, or it may be the final straw. The need to act in a professional way, given advantageous circumstances, thus may be what enables the nurse to get through this experience. On the other hand, the nurse's professional identity may itself complicate the pain of a patient's death—even where no particularly close nurse-patient relationship existed—by adding feelings of guilt and failure. The nurse's role, after all, is to save life and alleviate suffering. When it has not been possible to do either or both of these it is natural enough to ask why; and it is not unnatural, sometimes, to be less than rational about one's own possible errors or omissions.

The death of a patient may be difficult then because unfinished emotional business concerning a particular patient has to be worked through, or because anything less than a 'good' or timely death may create a sense of guilt and failure among professionals. The death of a patient may also be disturbing moreover when, for whatever reason, it brings home to those around a profound awareness of finality—that this is something no-one can do anything whatever to alter. This knowledge, and with it the awareness of our own mortality and finite powers, is difficult for many of us to come to terms with, because one measure of our achievement as people is the capacity to live in the past and the future as well as the present. In the face of death however, the past—much of which was preserved in the brain now dead—becomes much more tenuous, dependent now on the memories of others; while the present is empty and the future—for the dead person at least—no longer exists. Some way of working through this experience, it is true, may be found by many people in religion, while for others the experience may provide the impetus to different kinds of action. But the realisation of finality and finitude, when a particular death evokes it, does need to be worked through in some way which provides a tolerable and sustaining equilibrium between accepting this realisation and straining against it.

There are a variety of reasons, then, why the death of a particular patient may evoke strong emotional feelings, which need to be worked through, in a particular nurse. If the deaths of all patients evoked such feelings, or if all nurses responded to one death in this way, professional nursing care of the patient, his relatives and other patients would not be possible. But if no such feelings were ever evoked nurses would be less than human, rather than superhuman. The extent to which an individual nurse resists or allows herself to demonstrate an overt expression of her feelings when these are evoked may be a matter of personal and professional moral choice. But sometimes tears are inevitable and sometimes, when a whole ward has been aware of what has been happening behind the screens, it may be comforting to patients to know that nurses care, provided that this does not cast doubts on their competence. From the patient's point of view, clearly, evidence that the medical and nursing staff have 'failed' in another patient's case may be disturbing. For this reason it is understandable, when a patient has died in the night for example, that other patients, on asking where the patient is, may be told by a nurse that 'he has been moved to another part of the hospital'. There are moral pressures on both sides of the argument here, although, if evasion is chosen, the case for not telling the whole truth probably needs to be argued rather than assumed—as it could more easily have been in the paternalistic past. Similarly, there may be good reasons for not giving information about a patient's death over the telephone to enquirers outside the immediate family, when there is doubt whether all the family yet know, or whether they have had time to assimilate the knowledge. Related considerations also apply to summoning the family of a patient who may have died sooner than was expected. In subsequently breaking the news of a patient's death to his family, the way in which the truth is told is clearly as important as what is told.

When junior nurses ask how they should manage and what they should say and do when confronted with dying patients, the fact of death, and shocked relatives, they are often told 'You will know what to say and do when it happens.' This however is not always the case: nowadays the first dying patient encountered by a first year student may be the first dying person she has ever encountered, and the experience of having to touch a dead human body may be something for which she is completely unprepared. Whether there are any adequate ways in which students can be prepared for such experiences is doubtful: there is in the end no substitute for the real thing. Nor is there any way of avoiding the feelings of pain, grief, guilt and helplessness which can be evoked in encounters with the dying, with death and with those who are left. Under these circumstances the moral pressure to put a brave face on things must usually, for practical reasons, be heeded. But there are occasions when it cannot and perhaps should not be, for the very good reason that some overt expression of her own human fallibility and frailty may be required to help the individual nurse recognise and accept her feelings of pain, grief, guilt and helplessness in the face of death. For without such recognition and acceptance, feelings of this kind may be buried and denied, so that in the future either they resurface in irrational and inappropriate ways which are difficult to control, or, if they are controlled, can only be done so by a deadening in the nurse of those sensitivities to herself and to other people which are essential for good nursing care.

3

Responsibility and accountability in nursing

Nurses form an occupational group which provides a wide variety of services within society. As such, nursing has organised itself into a bureaucratic style of working which places individual nurses within a formal structure. This structure determines, to a large extent, the behaviour of the individual nurse: it puts limits upon her range of activities; and it holds her accountable for her actions both as an individual and as a member of the occupational group.

The organisational structure of nursing raises several issues which are pertinent to ethical debate about nursing. These issues can be divided into at least three areas: issues concerned with the nurse as a part of the nursing hierarchy; issues concerned with the nurse and other members of the health care team; and issues related to the nurse's responsibility to her own profession. In order to understand many of the difficulties which nurses confront in their day to day work it may be helpful to begin by examining the hierarchical structure of nursing, and then to discuss the other two areas mentioned.

The nursing structure

The nursing service, unlike medicine, is organised according to the principles of line management. Essentially, this means that qualified nurses, from the grade of staff nurse upwards, are organised into hierarchical grades within which each nurse is responsible for certain work and accountable to a senior nurse 'up the line'. Clearly, this is potentially a formalised system for 'buck-passing'. On the other hand, the system does not relieve the individual nurse of responsibility for her own actions. We shall return to this point later.

Today's nursing organisation is, in general terms, a development of the Nightingale tradition which itself was established upon principles borrowed from military organisation; and something of the military tradition has obviously been retained in titles such as 'nursing officer'. The organisation for the delivery of nursing care instituted by Florence Nightingale was designed in order to allow for a wide range of ability within the service, and it worked as long as obedience of the military kind prevailed. As Carpenter[1] puts it: 'The beauty of this idea lay in its simplicity, serving in turn to unify the occupation into a single community stretching from the lowest ranking nurse to the highest ranking nurse. The crucial element in the situation was the power of the matron.'

This early band of nurse managers, matrons, by insisting upon obedience from their nurses, achieved a nursing service which would follow doctors' orders unquestioningly, yet which would not allow itself to be disciplined by doctors. The nursing service came under the direct control of the matrons. In the 1960s, the Salmon and Mayston reorganisations replaced the matrons with a line management structure. This new structure resulted from Salmon's implicit call for an industrial model of professionalised management. Nursing was to be managed as might be any other workforce whose business it was to accomplish a task by means of group effort. The line management approach took the power which the old-style matrons held and shared it, to some extent, 'down the line' by giving different 'ranks' appropriate area of responsibility and making them accountable for their work to an immediate superior.

This new bureaucratic mode of operation poses problems for an occupational group which claims to be a profession. Autonomy and control over one's work are important hallmarks of a profession. Nursing has severe problems in this direction, not only because of the presence of the dominant profession of medicine, but also because the bureaucratic line management approach threatens to stifle professional judgement on the part of the individual nurse. The medical profession gets around this difficulty by operating a collegial approach, which accepts each doctor as a professional who gives and seeks advice among colleagues, and is open to judgement by his peers, but who is not held accountable for his day-to-day work to a management hierarchy. This difference in the organisational structures of medicine and nursing clearly presents problems when consultation and co-operation are required between individuals from the two professions.

As well as the military influence on nursing there was, of course, an even earlier religious influence. The older meaning of 'profession' has to do with the vows taken or 'professed' by members of religious orders, some of whom were responsible for the care of the sick and poor in mediaeval hospitals or hospices. These vows included obedience, which also was stressed in the military model, together with a strong sense of hierarchy. The religious model, too, emphasised the idea of the professed individual as a servant of others. This service emphasis was continued in Florence Nightingale's time. Nursing was not to be undertaken primarily for profit or financial gain. In practice, of course, nineteenth-century nursing seems to have been a means of providing work for the unmarriageable daughters of the middle and upper-middle classes. But the religious origins of its ideals also held out the promise of work which provided some measure of social worth. In this connection, the introduction of a capitalist rationality, which Salmon brought to the organisation of nursing, marks a further move away from its religious origins.

The nurse in the hierarchy

The underlying rationale of the line management structure on which the Salmon and Mayston reorganisations were based provides a key to understanding the power and authority structures of nursing. Provision was made within the reorganisation for the inclusion of grades below that of nursing officer, as is evidenced by the number 7 being attached to that grade, leaving lower numbers for lower grades. Although the line below ward sister has never been formalised, as it has above, the implicit hierarchical organisation from the most junior learner to the ward sister is obvious enough. In day-to-day practice on the wards the first year learner will take an order from a second year, as will a second year learner from a third year. From the very first days of training, learners are made aware of the fact that they are the newest recruits; and as soon as another group arrives they immediately feel that they have moved a rung up the ladder. From these early days therefore, a sense of the authority structure is acquired, even at the unofficial end of the hierarchy.

At this junior end of the line, line management principles are also recognised in other aspects of day-to-day practice. On any ward a senior nurse is recognised to be 'in charge'; during the daytime this nurse will almost certainly be qualified and is frequently the sister. With the shorter working week however, the sister can work only five of the fourteen daytime shifts; staff nurses and enrolled nurses will thus be 'in charge' for the remaining nine. On night duty, however, a student nurse is very likely to be left 'in charge' of a ward, with recourse to a night charge nurse who will be covering several wards. The remainder of the nurses on duty will take their work directives from the person who is in charge and will be accountable to that person for the work they are carrying out. Since there are a variety of ways in which patient care can be organised—in terms of 'who does what on this shift'—the nature of this organisation will have implications for the degree of responsibility and accountability which the individual nurse has.

Crucial to the functioning of this hierarchical organisation is an understanding by all nurses of the routines and 'hospital ways' of carrying out nursing and handling situations which arise in the course of nursing work. Nurses, that is, are made aware not only of their responsibilities in patient care, but also of the manner in which they should conduct themselves within the nursing hierarchy. Within this routinised, hierarchical structure, the individual has to learn how to cope with her personal values and to make decisions about her actions as a nurse.

Advantages and disadvantages

The hierarchical system of line management has certain obvious advantages. One advantage is that it brings some power of decision making closer to the area of patient care. A ward sister, for example, instead of having to ask the highest ranking nurse for extra help on a busy shift, might simply ask her immediate superior, the nursing officer, with whom she is in closer contact. On the other hand, requests involving greater changes may have to go to a higher authority 'up the line', while policy decisions may come 'down the line' through the nursing officer to the ward sister, who has to put policy into practice whether or not she finds it acceptable.

This form of management, then, puts the nurse in a position where she is not always able to act in the way in which she, as an individual, might see fit. Depending upon the circumstances, this can be a positive or a negative feature of the hierarchical organisation of nursing. If, for example, the nurse involved is inexperienced, or a learner, actions based on her own judgement might not be for the best. In such a case the hierarchical system and the restrictions it places upon the individual's behaviour may have advantages. For example:

A young patient decides that he is tired of waiting around the medical ward for the results of his tests and, despite his quite severe symptoms of a yet unknown cause, makes up his mind to take his own discharge. He waits until a quiet period in the afternoon when sister has gone for her break and only junior nurses are in evidence on the ward. A junior nurse sees him dressing and he tells her he is leaving. He is very articulate, telling her that he fully understands his condition and has every right to leave. The junior nurse knows that she should tell a qualified member of staff, in the hope that they might be able to persuade the patient that it is in his own interest to stay. On the other hand, as an individual she can see his point: she feels moreover that he is a sensible young man who would get in touch with his GP if he deteriorated in any way. Nevertheless, she follows the hospital-dictated procedure and, recognising that dealing with this situation falls outside her competence, she informs the staff nurse.

In this example, the advantage of the hierarchical organisation of nursing is that it affords protection to a less experienced member of staff. The junior nurse might well have thought that there would be no harm in simply letting the patient go—as indeed he had a legal as well as a moral right to do. However, as a nurse she was expected to follow hospital policy, which dictated that she should inform a senior nurse and that the patient must be required to sign himself out in the presence of nurses, who in turn must sign as witnesses of his discharge. In the event of the patient thus leaving the hospital of his own will, the student would not necessarily feel that she had compromised her own values, or indeed the patient's, since he had achieved his end. What, though, if he had been persuaded by senior staff to stay? The student nurse might then have felt a sense of guilt at having let him down by not following her own instincts. As an individual she might have liked to see him go: at the very least she might have wanted to see his right to choose respected. But as a nurse she would be concerned with his interests as well as his rights, and in the conflict between rights and interests, she might well have felt that it would be in his best interests to stay. In this case the practical solution was arrived at in terms of the student's position in the nursing hierarchy: she passed responsibility 'up the line'. Having done so, however, she still has to come to terms with the fact that had it not been for her action the patient might well have got his own way.

Conscientious objections

This example illustrates some of the difficulties involved when the nurse's personal view of the patient's best interests conflicts with the official view which the nurse is expected to follow. These difficulties are particularly acute if the nurse feels that she really must stand out against the official line, since if she loses the support of her colleagues she places herself in a very vulnerable position. In this connection the saying about there being safety in numbers is particularly true when it comes to making decisions about other people's lives.

There is, however, a further difficulty which may arise when a nurse decides to stand by her personal beliefs and perhaps refuse to participate in certain kinds of treatment, or in a particular treatment for one patient. This difficulty lies in the pressure the nurse's action places on those who do not exercise the right to abstain. One of the most obvious examples of this is the nurse's right not to participate in abortions. In the theatre this is a reasonably straightforward administrative problem, since only those nurses willing (or not objecting) to work with abortion lists will be employed there, although in a general theatre list this can still create difficulties for the staff who are left to cope after the conscientious objectors have absented themselves. But the issue is becoming increasingly problematic for nurses when abortions are being carried out on the wards. The clauses of the 1967 Abortion Act do not allow for nurses refusing to participate in the pre- or post-operative care of a patient having an abortion. What then is the position of the nurse in the care of a patient undergoing an induced abortion on the ward? Perhaps she might, reasonably, refuse to have anything to do with the administration of the drug. But what does she do when the patient requires help when vomiting as a result of the abortion-inducing drugs? It seems unlikely that a nurse would refuse to help a patient in such distress, but this does point up the limitations on the nurse's right to follow her own conscience in this situation. One practical way out of such a problem might be to carry out ward-situated abortions only in areas where learners are not required to work—trained staff, clearly, can choose where they might work. This solution, however, might open the way for a rather different kind of abortion service entering the health service, which might develop in a way not necessarily in the interests either of patients or of staff.

The underlying dilemma in the above discussion of the right of the nurse to opt out of abortion work is that if one nurse will not undertake certain work to which patients have a right, then another nurse must. A different aspect of this problem can be illustrated by a further example however.

A man of 27 with a wife and small daughter had hepatitis and renal failure. He had been on machine dialysis for three days a week. He was an in-patient, and although his progress was steady, it was not as good as was expected. The consultant decided that the dialysis machine could be used to better effect for other patients. A decision was therefore made to take the patient off the machine and to put him on diamorphine. This was done without much discussion and when the staff nurse was told to give the diamorphine injection she asked for time to discuss this with other staff. The nursing staff, except for the ward sister, decided to refuse to be involved with this injection because of the patient's age and his prognosis since coming off the dialysis machine and being given diamorphine. The night staff also refused. The night senior nurse, a third year student, was taken to the office and spoken to about her refusal, which upset her. Only the sister and the doctor gave the injection of diamorphine. The patient died before the next dialysis procedure was due.

This example illustrates the protection afforded by the hierarchy to the junior members of staff. However, it is also demonstrates that even when the junior nursing staff are prepared to stand together, they cannot always expect support from their seniors. In this case, had the ward sister taken the view of the majority of the nurses, then the doctors would have had to take both prescriptive and practical responsibility for their treatment. As it was, the senior nurses further up the line of management made the third year student feel very uncomfortable about the stance she took. This example clearly raises considerations on both sides of the argument. If nurses are to decide on conscientious grounds how far they are prepared to go along with certain forms of treatment, the carrying-out of patient care might well become a much more difficult matter than at present. Nursing still works very much according to the Nightingale promise that nurses will do as they are told. But as nurses become more vocal and aware of their rights, and patient care more fraught with ethical issues, the nursing service may well need to look again at its terms and conditions of employment. A hard line which states that all care undertaken in a particular hospital will be undertaken by all nurses clearly leaves the individual little scope for manoeuvre in moral matters. On the other hand, it would be administratively or operationally difficult to have a system of health care in which nurses could pick and choose among prescribed treatments.

Knowledge and control

Problems of a different kind again may be raised by the hierarchical structure of nursing when more junior members of staff have in fact more knowledge about a particular situation and are thus better suited to take relevant decisions. One example of this might be in an intensive care unit, where the sister in charge and her senior staff nurses may be in a better position than is the nursing officer to determine what staffing levels are required in the unit at any given time. The nursing officer may perhaps be out of touch with intensive care nursing, or may indeed never have had any clinical experience in the area. She is, nevertheless, in a position of authority which allows her to deploy staff in her unit as she sees fit. Even if this leaves the sister short-staffed, she has to defer to the decision of her senior.

At ward level also, the hierarchical order may require a more junior nurse to obey the instructions of a less well-informed senior. Learner nurses encounter this problem when they come across a ward where the nursing care being carried out does not conform to the 'correct practice' which they have been taught in the college of nursing. A typical example of the problem is in the treatment of patients' pressure areas. Some of the 'old school' approaches to preventive measures in skin care generally, and pressure area care in particular, have been shown to be not only ineffectual but possibly harmful. The learner nurse is faced with a difficult situation when a ward sister asks her to carry out a procedure for a patient which the nurse knows is not in the patient's best interest. The learner may well be able to cite the relevant research, to describe the preferred treatment and to justify her case. But the fact remains that she is an unqualified junior questioning her senior. The easiest practical solution to such a problem would probably be to go along with the sister's wishes. But what about the nurse's responsibility to her patient? There is also the question of litigation which, following the United States, is increasingly becoming a matter for consideration in Britain. Patients are more aware of their rights as consumers in the NHS than has been the case in the past. Legal proceedings can be instigated if patients or relatives feel that they have a case against the medical or nursing staff with respect to their treatment and care. If, then, the learner nurse has reason to believe that the care she is being asked by her seniors to give might be harmful to the patients, a confrontation with the senior nurse might seem the only course open to her. Such behaviour might not be consistent with the line of authority approach, but it might be morally and legally prudent in such a case.

Responsibility, ward organisation and record keeping

As has already been mentioned, the style of organisation on a ward can have implications for the amount of responsibility which an individual nurse carries. We can distinguish two main styles of ward organisation: one, commonly referred to as patient allocation, where the patient is the central focus; and one where tasks and routine are the main features. Patient allocation means that each nurse is assigned one or more patients and is responsible for their care. The use of detailed care plans, in which individualised instructions for the patient's care can be found, is a characteristic of this style of ward management. These care plans may also be used for the other style of organisation however, where they can be combined and translated into routine tasks in terms of the whole ward. In a patient allocation system, the individual nurse is responsible for all the care of one or more patients. In many ways this puts more pressure on the nurse than if she were simply part of the ward work-force with a share in the care of all patients. If the nurse knows that she is responsible simply for, say, fluids and fluid balance charts for the whole ward, then she can go about her day's 'tasks' in a fairly routine way without taking responsibility for any single patient: while she takes care of fluids, others in turn will attend to baths, dressings, recording and so forth for the same patients. Thus the patients, or at least their needs, are fragmented and distributed among the nurses, who have collective responsibility for the care: but the weight of the responsibility falls upon the nurse in charge who distributed the tasks.

One of the commonest arguments against patient allocation is that more staff are required to put it into practice. But in a recent study of student nurses' views on nursing,[2] a number of students stated a positive preference for routine and a task-centred approach because it represented a foolproof system for getting through the work without items of care being missed out. On these grounds it can be argued that the certainty which a routine provides can benefit the patients, who may rest assured that their basic needs will be met. Junior nurses also may gain security by avoiding the stress of being wholly responsible for any one patient. Against this view, however, must be set the possible therapeutic benefits of a patient-centred approach and its advantages in terms of work satisfaction for many nurses.

Whichever style of organisation is adopted, however, responsibility ultimately falls on one member or other of the nursing staff, whether it be the nurse wholly responsible for a particular patient or the nurse in charge of a task-oriented ward. In practice, of course, the nurse's employer, the health authority, is also vicariously responsible for her actions or omissions, and while individual nurses may be sued by patients or relatives along with the health authority, it is recognised that the latter is most likely to be able to pay any damages awarded by the court. On the other hand, it is worth noting that the employing authority is then entitled to try to recover its costs from the individual nurse.

In such circumstances, clearly, record-keeping is a crucial factor. If how the patient has been treated can be seen from accurate notes kept and signed by the nurses involved in the case, then, should there be any dispute, a statement of the facts is available. The kind of issues involved can be illustrated by an example.

An elderly patient, who was unable to walk, persisted in getting out of bed, unaided, during the night and repeatedly fell on the floor. Because of the layout of the ward and the lack of staff, constant observation was not possible. Cotsides were not used in the unit and extra sedation was not recommended. The accident forms often amounted to three a night, although not every night. The senior nursing officer questioned the number of forms and recommended that it was not necessary to fill these in at each incident, because of the frequency with which these falls occurred. The nurse who had been filling in the forms had then to ask herself whether she should continue to do so, to cover herself from the legal aspect, or whether she should carry out her senior's instructions.

In this case the records concerned—the hospital accident forms—were additional to the nursing care records. The senior nurse manager looked at the situation in terms of wasted time and effort: but the nurse who was most immediately involved was anxious to follow the hospital procedure, not least for her own protection.

The question of record-keeping is also relevant to recent cases of parents complaining about the lack of information received from health visitors in connection with advice on immunisation. There now seems to be some risk of a health visitor being sued for omitting to make parents aware of all the side effects and possible dangers associated with vaccination.[3] Health visitors, clearly, do not record every word of their information to clients, so that in court it could well be the client's word against the health visitor's. Here too a history of clear and full record-keeping would be in the health visitor's interest if such a case were to be brought.

The nurse and the health care team

In the context of the health care team, possibly the greatest scope for conflict is in the relationship between nursing and medical practice. Apart from any other differences between doctors and nurses, there are two structural reasons for this. One, already mentioned, is the difference between the collegial organisation of medicine and the hierarchical organisation of nursing. The collegial model is based upon professional trust, individual discretion and an informal system of regulation by one's peers: in practice, a junior doctor will seek advice from and be guided by his more experienced senior colleagues, but with much less need for a formal line of command than in nursing. At the ward level, this can create problems. If, for example, a registrar acts in some way which contravenes hospital policy, he enjoys greater freedom to do so than does the ward sister who is associated with this action. The registrar may, say, leave the ward and ask to be telephoned if a seriously ill patient's condition deteriorates. He may then find it prefectly acceptable to order a drug over the telephone, await the outcome and decide to return only if certain changes occur. This action may meet the approval of his colleagues, and the ward sister, as an individual, may consider it perfectly reasonable behaviour and go along with it, not least because the patient will benefit from receiving the drug sooner rather than having to wait for the doctor's return. However, the ward sister will also be aware that to order drugs over the telephone is against hospital policy, which she is supposed to implement, and that if she complies with the registrar's wishes she will not enjoy the support of her seniors. This is only one example of the kinds of conflict which arise when these two front-line professionals try to work together. At a day-to-day level both must be able to co-operate in planning the care of the patients: the smooth and efficient running of the ward depends very much on the working relationship between doctor and nurse at this level. The nursing staff however are to some extent hidebound by the rules involved in being the hospital's 'clinical civil service', and this brings them potentially into conflict with doctors who have more of the status of free agents who practise their craft in hospitals.

The second structural factor with potential for conflict in the nurse-doctor relationship lies in the nature of nursing as an occupation. Nursing can be said to be in part dependent upon and in part independent of medical practice. There are, clearly, some areas of nursing work which mostly have to do with carrying out the care prescribed by doctors. In this sense the nurse is simply following orders. There are however other areas of care, which mostly have to do with that patient's comfort and social well-being, in which the nurse should take action which is independent of medicine. Doctors have a tendency to see nursing as an entirely dependent profession, which exists to help them. Some nurses are happy to go along with this working definition. Others prefer to develop their nursing skills, arrive at decisions how best they think the patient might be cared for and form what we might call a nursing opinion. Having formed her opinion, the nurse might then wish to question the work of the doctor. At a more pragmatic than ethical level she might, for example, question the wisdom of his prescription. Often an experienced ward sister will be in a position to advise a more junior doctor upon the best treatment in cases of which she has had past experience. If the doctor is not prepared to listen to her opinion, or having listened ignores it, the nurse is then faced with the choice between letting the matter drop, possibly to the detriment of her patient on the grounds that 'the doctor knows best', or pressing her opinion to the extent of calling in a senior doctor or refusing to co-operate in the treatment. On the military analogy she may then marshall her troops and dictate to her staff what the nursing line will be. In the case of such confrontation, teamwork breaks down and both professions retreat to their respective managers and colleagues, while the issue moves from the pragmatic to the ethical. The determining factor in the outcome of such conflicts often lies in the answer to the question about 'who carries the can'. Nurses, to their own satisfaction, might have a right to a nursing opinion and also a right to challenge medical staff. But what of the responsibility? The 'contract' which the patient enters into when he is ill is between patient and doctor. The patient is thus ultimately the doctor's responsibility.

Difficulties of this kind are often most acute in areas such as geriatric medicine, terminal care, psychiatry and obstetrics where team decisions are often taken but where the responsibility is ultimately that of the doctor. Because of this, the teamwork ideal may be difficult to translate into practice. Further difficulties can be caused by the fact that health care professions and occupations other than medicine and nursing may each have their own hierarchies, lines of accountability. rules, regulations and working practices. Many decisions that directly affect the care of patients and the running of wards— from cleaning to hospital meals, portering to the ambulance service—are outside the control of the sister and her staff, however much patients and their relatives may imagine that they are responsible. In this context, as in relationships with doctors, the qualities of tact and diplomacy are a necessary part of the nurse's moral equipment.

Responsibility to the profession

Professional groups which enjoy a monopoly on the service they provide must also accept responsibility for their standards of practice. Nursing, as a professional group, is clearly concerned about its standards of care. One has only to look at the nursing press or reports from nursing conferences to see that a preoccupation with standards and the quality of patient care is one which many nurses share. Typically, the professions claim to have knowledge and skills which allow their members to give some form of service. The fact that the service is of a specialised nature with a theoretical base makes it difficult for the lay person to judge the performance of professionals. For this reason, the professions themselves seek to develop ways of assuring society that it will be protected from any undesirable consequences of the professional monopoly. To this end the profession sets its own standards of practice, trains its own recruits, disciplines its members and strives to maintain its standards. Clearly there are problems in a system by which the profession seeks to maintain its own standards. The arguments for this practice centre on the fact that a specialist knowledge is required to understand professional behaviour and so self-regulation is the most effective way to maintain standards. The difficulty, however, is that the closed nature of the professional organisation prevents any independent viewpoint being brought to bear on the profession's practice.

The fact that professionals are not above the law goes some way to alleviating any fears which society might have about professionals abusing their privileged position. The courts provide a means of regulating the conduct of professionals whose conduct moves outside the law. While the law may not be the most appropriate medium for resolving ethical issues, it does have the virtue of impartiality and can set limits to the harmful potential of monopoly power. On the other hand, while it would be undesirable to have a medical profession whose members were never required to justify their actions, the complexities of medical decision-making are such that a legalistic approach to a debate about its rights and wrongs may be unhelpful. For example:

A nurse as part of an intensive care team has been involved in the care of brain-damaged patient. After the patient has been on a respirator for a few days, the physicians establish that brain death has occurred. After discussion with the relatives and the nursing staff, the doctor in charge of the patient's case decides that the respirator should be turned off and the patient's heart left to stop. The whole team is in complete agreement with the decision and the nurse who has been looking after the patient turns off the machine.

If in such a case, circumstances for some reason lead to a court hearing because the life support machine has been switched off, the complex series of events which led up to switching off the machine might sound very different in a court room. The way in which evidence is handled often leaves little scope for an explanation of all the surrounding circumstances. Thus the description of events might be interpreted by a lay jury in a way very different from that of informed medical and nursing opinion. On the other hand again, is it not right that an outside view should be sought? Will a professional group not simply confirm its own conduct and because of familiarity fail to see the flaws in its practice which a lay person might see? Doubts of this kind, clearly, cannot be dismissed out of hand, not least because even when cases come to the courts the profession's own definition of events is very influential. As McCall Smith remarks, in his discussion of the legal aspects of the Rcn code,[4] 'the law may ultimately be called upon to define what is acceptable practice on the part of the professions but it tends to do so on the basis of what the professions themselves suggest. The law, then, looks for guidance to professional consensus, while the professions naturally look to the law for a statement of what they can or cannot do.'

In the light of this circular relationship between consensus and the law, McCall Smith concludes that 'the promulgation of a code of professional conduct is of major legal significance, in that it can be influential in the moulding of legal attitudes'.

From the profession's point of view also, codes of ethics or codes of conduct are important—both as ways of proclaiming publicly their trustworthiness and as means of giving their members some guide as to their practice. In this connection it is perhaps useful to think of a profession's standards on the one hand at a micro-level, in the sense of how individual members behave towards their patients, clients and colleagues, and on the other hand at a macro-level where the professional ethic can be seen as something which the whole profession upholds and which can be invoked by individual members to support their behaviour. Throughout this discussion the whole code of ethics at these two levels will be drawn upon.

Codes of ethics

There are several codes of ethics to which we might turn in order to gain some idea of their form and purpose. The medical profession in Britain has never had an agreed code, although the highly regarded but rarely read Hippocratic Oath serves as an 'ethical flag'. Nursing and social work have followed what they took to be a medical lead and produced their own codes of ethics. The practice of producing such codes is probably linked with the desire of certain occupations to claim professional status. It is interesting to note in passing that the British Sociological Association, for example, also recently felt the need to formulate a code of ethics.

By Florence Nightingale's Pledge, a nurse solemnly promised to 'pass my life in purity and to practise my profession faithfully. I will abstain from whatever is deleterious and mischievous and will not take or administer any harmful drug.' Since Florence Nightingale's time, various codes have been produced by the International Council of Nurses (1953, 1965, 1973); and in 1976 the Royal College of Nursing produced a discussion document entitled 'Code of Professional Conduct'. Before examining these nursing codes and the whole question of responsibility to the profession, it is worth considering in greater detail what we might expect from a code of ethics.

As has been said, British medicine has never in fact had agreed written code of ethics, although the code of ethics adopted by the American Medical Association in 1848 was based on an earlier code drawn up by the Manchester physician Thomas Percival.[5] Subsequent written codes have tended to be the result of a fear of a decline, or an actual decline, in medical standards, or a response to a particular ethical debate. The 1947 Nuremberg Code, concerned with permissible medical experiments, for example, was drawn up after revelations about Nazi war crimes involving medical experiments on human subjects. Further examples drawn up by the World Medical Association include: the Declaration of Geneva (1948 and 1968), an updated version of the Hippocratic Oath; the Declaration of Helsinki (1964 and 1975) on research involving

human subjects; the Declaration of Sydney (1968) on determination of the time of death; the Declaration of Oslo (1970)
on therapeutic abortion; and the Declaration of Tokyo (1975)
on torture and degrading treatment or punishment. Ethical
guidelines for psychiatrists were also drawn up by the World
Psychiatric Association in the Declaration of Hawaii (1977).[6]

To illustrate the uses and limitations of such ethical codes,
let us examine just one part of the Declaration of Oslo, on
therapeutic abortion, which states (Clause 6) that 'If a doctor
considers that his convictions do not allow him to advise or
perform an abortion, he may withdraw while ensuring the
continuity of (medical) care by a qualified colleague.'

At first sight this clause appears to provide a fairly straightforward guideline which the doctor might follow. It makes
certain actions possible for the doctor and allows him a
conscience clause to get out of undertaking a practice which
is against his principles. It does however leave the potential
for practical difficulties. If no such colleague is available
(either, say, in a routine case or if his colleagues are equally
opposed to abortion) can the individual doctor expect to work
according to his beliefs if these are at variance with those of
many of his patients?

In practice then, codes of ethics clearly have their limitations
and cannot be seen as always providing the answer to day-to-
day moral dilemmas. What such codes can do, however, is to
set out the general values and policies to which professional
practice is supposed to conform. As such, they provide a
means of laying down standards of conduct which a profession
might expect its members to meet. Indeed, in the Rcn discussion document, this is recognised. The introduction states that[7]
'no code can do justice to every individual case and therefore
that any set of principles must remain constantly open to discussion both within the nursing profession and outside it.' The
same document supplies a further reason for ethical codes
when it states that codes should serve to 'provide a clear and
comprehensive document for further discussion, particularly
during training.'

The code thus states the 'ideal' professional standards in a
clear way which can be recognised as a description of the
desired behaviour of professionals. If, as an individual, a nurse
is unsure of the position that she should adopt in some situ-

ation, the code can supply some guidance. For example, if a nurse is unhappy about a particular treatment which a dying patient is receiving, she might feel that as an individual she has no option other than to follow the doctor's instructions. She does, however, have not only the right, but also the duty to express her opinion about the effect of treatment on her patients. While a nurse might feel diffident about making her opinion known, especially if she is expressing views which run counter to those of the doctor who is prescribing the care, she can find support for her action in the codes of ethics. The Rcn code, for example, states that [8] 'Measures which jeopardise the safety of patients, such as unnecessary treatment, hazardous experimental procedures and the withdrawal of professional services during employment disputes should be actively opposed by the profession as a whole.' The individual nurse then must live up to this code and express opinions when she has them. She can be said to have a duty to her profession to behave in such a way, even though the organisation within which she works historically gives more weight to doctors' opinions.

Responsibility for professional standards

If nurses are to be accountable for their care in a professional sense they also have a duty to keep up to date in the knowledge base of their profession. It is not sufficient that a nurse pass her final examinations, qualify and then never consider it necessary to continue her education. Nurses must be responsible for the care they give, and it cannot be claimed that because nurses work according to doctors' orders they are exempt from any responsibility. For example, if a nurse thinks that a doctor's prescription contains the wrong dose of the drug she has a duty to question it and, if she is still in doubt, to refuse to give the drug. A nurse, along with the doctor, might be charged with negligence, for instance, if she failed to recognise the incorrectly prescribed dosage of a commonly known drug such as digoxin.

One might, of course, argue that it is the doctor's business to get the prescription right and that the nurse cannot be held responsible. However, the nurse takes responsibility for her actions and must carry out her patient care in an intelligent way which includes recognising potential harm to her patients. Again, from a code of ethics, this time from the ICN (1973), 'The nurse takes appropriate action to safeguard the individual when his care is endangered by a co-worker or any other person.' The general point about responsibility for professional standards is also made by the Rcn code.[9] 'The professional authority of nurses is based upon their training and experience in day-to-day care of ill persons at home or in hospital; and the enhancement of positive health in the community at large. All members of the nursing profession have a responsibility to continue to develop their knowledge and skill in these matters.'

In order to maintain professional standards, then, nurses must inform themselves of advances in knowledge of nursing care. Not only must the profession ensure that its new recruits achieve a certain standard before they are allowed to practise; but it must also make certain that its established members maintain those standards. Indeed, because nurse training involves a substantial amount of learning 'on the job', it is imperative that practitioners keep themselves up to date so that the learners are exposed to practice of the right standard.

Practice which is based on sound principles and established empirical evidence might distinguish a professional from a lay approach to activity in a given field. At a macro-level the profession must ensure that its standards of practice are supported by a sound theoretical base. At a more individual or micro-level, the practitioners must be sure that they are aware of the latest advances in the discipline and that their practice is up to date.

In the case of nursing, much of the work which nurses undertake was for a long time, and in some instances still is, based upon tradition rather than research. However for some years now nursing research has been undertaken and its findings made available to the profession. This means that the individual nurse can no longer plead ignorance if she chooses to follow tradition rather than a proven form of treatment. A good example of this, which we have already mentioned, is the care and treatment of pressure areas and sores. Even after publication of findings to the contrary,[10] nurses continued to rub soap and water, spirit and a variety of other doubtful applications on patients' skin. For a learner nurse this particular example might pose ethical difficulties. From the college of nursing she will have been supplied with the latest research-based information in relation to the care of pressure areas; yet on the ward she could be told that the sister's policy involves a treatment which the student knows has been shown to be harmful. Given that a nurse is supposed to be not only responsible for her actions but also morally accountable for them, this student's choice between following the teachings of the college and obeying the ward sister is a difficult one. In this particular example, because of the workings of the nursing hierarchy, it might also be hard for the student to invoke the professional code of practice in defence of her disregarding the sister's instructions.

Clearly the macro professional level and the micro individual level converge at some point and share responsibility for advancing the knowledge of the discipline. Accurate and meaningful record-keeping on the part of the nurse can provide the data required to evaluate present practice. Thus, whilst each individual nurse will not be a researcher as such, she should take a responsible attitude towards her nursing record-keeping in order that the effects of X upon Y in nursing care can be documented. The nursing process is an attempt at such an approach to nursing. For example, toileting practices with elderly incontinent patients could be recorded carefully, and after a period the success of individual programmes could be assessed in terms of the degree of continence attained. Nurses might take a lead from their medical colleagues in this respect. Doctors do not all follow identical treatment patterns with patients with similar conditions. For instance, coronary care might vary from one doctor to the next with equally successful results. It matters little that the treatments are different; what does matter, however, is that doctors take note of the effects of their treatment and thus build up a working repertoire of medical practice, based, of course, upon the theory available to all those practising medicine but refined according to their observations. Further, if a doctor arrives at a particularly successful way of treating a condition, he will communicate this to his colleagues through the professional journals.

Being morally responsible for one's actions, of course, can be a stressful business. A nurse will often be involved in team decisions and have the support of her colleagues, but she is still both legally accountable and morally responsible for her own actions. This involves accepting the uncertainty and distress which might go along with these actions. To quote again from the Rcn discussion document,[11] 'nurses are in a unique position to observe the condition of the patient at all hours of the night and day and have received basic intruction in drug dosages, effects of treatment etc. For this reason they are morally obliged to question medical instructions which they believe will cause the patient harm or unnecessary distress, even though they may fear adverse effects on their career from doing so.'

Reporting on colleagues

Aside from having a personal individual responsibility for their own practice and maintenance of professional standards, nurses also have a wider responsibility to the nursing profession. This means that they should be prepared to report poor standards of care, and nursing which is not practised in accordance with the professional standard, when they encounter it. This presents perhaps the most trying moral difficulties of all.

If poor practice is to be curbed it must be reported and it is a fact of life that often the person best placed to observe and report bad practice on the part of a nurse will be another nurse. What price professional loyalty then? If a nurse sees one of her colleagues maltreating a patient, for example an elderly patient or a mentally handicapped person, what is she to do? Her own private morality will tell her that what she saw was wrong and that the correct line of action would be to report the incident. Still at an individual level the nurse might feel something of a 'sneak' telling tales about another individual's action. Yet she is likely to be able to squash this fear because of the rights of the maltreated patient whose position she is really defending. She then has the profession to contend with. The colleague has brought disgrace upon the profession to which she belongs. Nurses are trusted by patients, indeed by society as a whole, to be caring and kind. They are put in a position of trust by virtue of having the care and in many senses the charge of the lives of other individuals. The nurse who witnesses a colleague's malpractice is then faced with a choice between exposing the colleague and risking publicity and the damage to the professional image which goes with it, and keeping quiet, hence betraying the patient's trust.

If the nurse faced with this choice is a learner then the dilemma is more acute. For, aside from the conflict of loyalty towards the profession and loyalty to the trust of patients she has her own future career as a nurse to consider. As Beardshaw[12] points out, 'are nurses able to protect their patients' interests by speaking up when they are abused? . . . often they are not. They may be forced to stand by when individual patients are ill-treated or when poor conditions deprive them of adequate care. Their silence is enforced by feelings of impotence, and by fears of reprisals. The victimisation of some nurses who have spoken up about abuse is a vivid illustration that these fears can be well founded.'

If a nurse is going to complain about the conduct of another nurse, then, she has to consider whether she will be listened to, believed, what it will do to her other relationships within the hospital and ultimately her career prospects. Even though it might be a patient's suffering which is at stake it is a difficult thing to (as Beardshaw puts it) 'blow the whistle' on one's colleagues. One D.N.E's comment[13] sums it up: 'Students still comment as follows: "we would get told off for interfering"; "no-one would take any notice of me"; "I need a job in the future". All worry about victimisation.'

Beardshaw points up the difficulties which exist in interpreting the ICN code of nursing ethics in terms of student nurses. She asks how the nurse can follow the ICN code and take 'appropriate action to safeguard the individual when his care is endangered by a co-worker or any other person' when she is subject to both the medical profession and the nursing hierarchy. And she concludes[14] that the position of the student nurse 'encapsulates an essential contradiction of nursing professionalism—"a profession waiting for orders", where emphasis on obedience to authority dilutes the professional responsibility of individual nurses.'

NOTES AND REFERENCES

1. Carpenter M 1977 The new managerialism and professionalism in nursing. In: Stacey M et al Health and the division of labour, Croom Helm, London

2. Melia K M 1981 Student nurses' accounts of their work and training: a qualitative analysis. Unpublished Ph D thesis, University of Edinburgh
3. Whincup M 1981 The duties of a health visitor. Nursing Times 77(13): 567–568; and Saunders G 1981 Parents of 'brain damage' boy claim £250 000. The Scotsman, October 8.
4. Royal college of nursing code of professional conduct 1976. Journal of Medical Ethics 3(3): 122.
5. Leake C D 1975 Percival's medical ethics, Robert E Krieger Publishing Company, New York.
6. Duncan A S, Dunstan G R, Welbourn R B 1981 Declarations. In: Dictionary of medical ethics, rev. edn. Darton, Longman & Todd, London
7. Royal college of nursing code of professional conduct 1976. Journal of Medical Ethics 3(3): 115
8. Royal college of nursing code of professional conduct 1976. Journal of Medical Ethics 3(3): 117
9. Royal college of nursing code of professional conduct 1976. Journal of Medical Ethics 3(3): 117
10. Norton D 1975 Research and the problem of pressure sores. Nursing Times 140: 65–67
11. Royal college of nursing code of professional conduct 1976. Journal of Medical Ethics 3(3): 118
12. Beardshaw V 1981 Conscientious objectors at work, Social Audit, London, p 2
13. Beardshaw V 1981 Conscientious objectors at work, Social Audit, London, p 57.
14. Beardshaw V 1981 Conscientious objectors at work, Social Audit, London, p 56

4

Moral dilemmas in direct nurse/patient relationships

The rights of patients

So far we have considered nursing ethics largely from the standpoint of the individual nurse or of the nurse in her relationship with her colleagues. Now, however, we must turn to the consideration of a number of moral dilemmas which relate directly to the nurse's responsibility in the care of patients. In real life a moral dilemma is a situation where the nurse is forced to make a difficult (and often painful) choice between conflicting moral obligations knowing that none of the available options is really satisfactory or ideal. The main types of recurrent moral dilemma may be grouped under four headings:

(a) Confidentiality and telling the truth to patients or relatives
(b) Deciding between therapeutic and palliative treatment
(c) Setting limits to the control and direction of patients
(d) Balancing the rights of patients and the interests of third parties.

Moral dilemmas of these kinds raise fundamental questions about the *rights* of patients and the scope and limits of the nurse's *responsibility*. The term 'rights' and the term 'responsibility' are always closely linked to one another and both have connections with another fundamental moral term, namely 'justice'. When we say that a person has rights we mean that he has a claim on other people, that other people have a responsibility to help him achieve his rights and to protect his rights from violation. But rights are not private to individuals. Moral and legal rights are common to all men. Your rights are not absolute because they are limited by my rights. We can assist one another to achieve our rights, we can help to protect one another's rights, but we also limit one another's rights. This is where justice comes into it. Issues of justice are involved not only when someone is denied their rights but when someone demands and exercises their rights at the expense of others. If we claim moral and legal rights we must also accept corresponding responsibility for one another and be willing to be accountable to others.

The first two of these areas of moral dilemma are more personal, in the sense that the individual patient's rights are most important in deciding what ought to be done. In the second two classes of moral dilemma the rights of others and the common good take on a greater importance and have to be taken into account in setting limits to the rights of patients. We shall discuss the first two in this chapter and the second pair in Chapter 5.

The specific rights of patients flow from the kind of relationship into which they enter with health-care staff. When the patient is lucid, ambulant and able to approach the health services independently for help there is a kind of contract set up in which the patient agrees to co-operate in investigations, treatment and rehabilitation, in return for appropriate medical care and treatment. The situation is rather different if the patient is brought in unconscious, or is unconsultable because of the specific nature of his disease or injury or by reason of insanity. Here the health-professionals have to assume total responsibility for the patient and must fall back on their own and their professional moral code for guidance. A third situation is one where the doctor or nurse is involved with the patient as a friend—either through previous association, special circumstances of shared confidences, or because the patient is dying and needs care and support rather than therapy. Here the relationship may take on a more intimate form and the moral commitment in the contractual relationship may need to be re-negotiated as something more personal and informal.

The ordinary situation which we described first takes the form of an implicit or explicit *contract* in which reciprocal rights and duties (or responsibilities) are recognised. In the second case, governed by *code*, the professional exercises responsibility on behalf of the patient. In the third kind of situation we need a different term to describe the new kind of relationship which develops through deepening trust and friendship between the provider of care and the person receiving the care. The term *covenant* has been suggested for this because the patient may feel able to make unusual demands and have these respected and the professional may be prepared to make special sacrifices and to act 'over and above the call of duty'.[1]

In terminal care the balance of power between patient and caring professional changes with changes in the independence or helplessness of the patient. This means that the balance of rights and responsibilities in the caring relationship changes correspondingly. At different stages it may be appropriate to think of the relationship more in terms of code or covenant than in terms of contract, but it is useful to begin by considering what is implied in the contract to care.

There are three basic rights of patients which flow directly from the nature of the Doctor/Patient contract (or more generally from the contract of the patient with the health services). These rights are:

The Right to Know
The Right to Privacy
The Right to Treatment.

Every patient has the *right to be adequately informed* about his condition and its proposed management—about his diagnosis, treatment and prognosis. Every patient has a *right to privacy*, in the sense of being entitled to respect for the dignity of his person and the privacy of confidential information he shares with medical or nursing staff. Every patient, who is taken on as a patient, has a *right to treatment*—a right to expect that he will be cared for and that those who care for him will do him no harm.[2]

However, two things need to be said about these rights: first, that they are not absolute; and, second, that an individual patient while having these rights may choose not to exercise his rights. The right to know is not absolute because it is part of the responsibility of the caring professional to decide in the best interests of the patient how, when and how much to tell. The patient too may decide that he does not want to discuss the details of his condition with the medical or nursing staff. He has in a sense a right not to know. The right to privacy is not absolute because the demands of caring for others in similar need may require that patients sacrifice some of their privacy, for example, on entering a public ward. Where team management of patients is necessary confidentiality may have to be extended in the sense of sharing relevant information with other members of the team in the interests of better patient care. Similarly some patients may be very concerned about their right to privacy, others may not be bothered. The right to treatment, which is both a moral right arising from the doctor's agreement to take you on as a patient, and a legal right (in the UK) following from the legislation by which the NHS was set up, is nevertheless not an absolute right because resources are not unlimited and the needs of other patients also have to be considered. Further, the patient has a right (recognised in law) to refuse treatment. When treatment is forced on him against his will this constitutes an assault and the patient is entitled (unless he is certified insane) to sue for damages. Even the right to refuse treatment is not morally speaking an absolute right and the courts may uphold the doctor's right to give treatment against the patient's wishes where he considers this is in the best interests of the patient (e.g. in giving life-saving blood transfusions to an injured Jehovah's Witness).

The interpretation of rights and duties in any specific situation always involves sensitivity to the unique circumstances and needs of individuals as well as discriminating judgement based on wide practical experience of similar situations. The resolution of moral dilemmas, where there is a clear conflict of rights or duties, is never easy. It demands a willingness to negotiate the best solution possible to safeguard the rights of all or alternatively to seek the solution which compromises least the rights of all concerned. This task may demand Solomonic wisdom in practice and the individual nurse or doctor may well have to take riskful and painful decisions knowing full well that the solution is far from ideal and may actually be wrong. Learning to accept the guilt for less-than-perfect decisions is part of learning what responsibility is all about.

Confidentiality and telling the truth to patients or relatives

Consider the dilemma of a young staff nurse in a paediatric hospital:

> Mary, aged 13 years, was admitted with acute myeloid leukaemia. Over the next two and a half years she was in and out of hospital at increasingly frequent intervals. The permanent ward staff established a good relationship with Mary and her family during this period. Initially her parents did not accept the diagnosis, but with much support and reassurance eventually accepted the situation fairly well.
>
> Two and a half years after the first admission, Mary was admitted for terminal care. Throughout the course of her illness her parents had been adamant that Mary should not be told what was wrong with her. This was still the situation when Mary was admitted for the last time. We tried to point out to her parents that Mary was no longer a child and that if the question of her condition arose, it might help her to know the truth, but they still refused to let her be told.
>
> Three days before she died, Mary asked outright if she was going to die. She said she felt she was getting worse rather than better, and she asked directly what it was like to die.
>
> In spite of her parents' views I felt that I had to be truthful with Mary as she was no longer a child but 15½ years old. We talked about death and I explained to her that everyone had to die sooner or later. I was with her when she died, as were her parents, and she died peacefully and calmly. I felt I had done the right thing in telling her, but felt that I had betrayed her parents' trust, which had been built up over nearly three years.

Would you have told Mary that she was dying? Do you believe Mary's parents had a right to forbid the nursing staff to tell her the truth about her condition? If you agree that Mary should have been told, when do you think she should have been told and by whom?

We have argued that patients generally have a *right to know*. When they enter into a contract with the doctor or health services for care and treatment, part of what is involved is a necessary sharing of truth. The patient is expected to answer the doctor's questions, to allow him to make a physical examination, to undertake tests and investigations. The patient exposes himself to intimate physical and psychological examination including investigation of his social circumstances. In return for sharing this information about himself with the doctor (and other members of the caring team) the patient is entitled to expect to be told the truth about his condition— including the doctor's diagnosis, proposed course of treatment, and the likely outcome. As a vulnerable individual, in need of help, who has entrusted himself to the care of doctors and nurses, he is also entitled to expect that his confidences will be respected.

Truth-sharing cannot be separated from confidentiality, because truth-sharing is a matter of trust and willingness to carry some responsibility for the truth shared. Only a cynical or irresponsible individual will 'tell the truth and be damned'. Keeping secrets is a way of protecting people who have made themselves vulnerable by sharing their secrets with you. Not telling someone the truth or keeping secrets from them may be a way of protecting them too. Often we hesitate to tell people the truth (when the truth is painful) because we are unwilling or unable to accept the full responsibility which truth-sharing entails. Sharing with someone the fact that they are dying is not only a painful experience, but may be a costly one in terms of the time and emotional energy required to support them as they come to terms with reality. Truth-sharing means sharing the pain and grief, anger and despair that knowing the truth may cause. If there is not a context of well-established understanding, trust and caring, if there is no possibility that you can provide continuing support to the individual concerned, then 'telling them the truth' may be a cruel and irresponsible thing to do.

The staff nurse in this case recognised that knowing the truth that Mary was dying imposed certain responsibilities on her, to protect Mary's vulnerability (a feeling she shared with Mary's parents), but she also recognised that Mary had a right to know the truth. The dilemma she faced was the conflict of loyalties to Mary and her parents because of the trust and understanding that had grown up between her and Mary on the one hand and between her and the parents on the other. The problem was made more difficult by her uncertainty that it was right to tell Mary and her sense of guilt at going against the declared wishes of her parents. She may also have been aware of having been specially chosen by Mary as the one to ask this momentous question. Was it not possible that the distraught parents, faced with losing their daughter, were using the staff nurse in a vain attempt to reassert their rights over their daughter? In such a situation which does the nurse put first: the rights of the parents or the rights of the patient?

In this connection some general observations may be relevant. The policy of openness adopted by hospices for the dying is based not only on the belief that the patient has a right to know (particularly if he asks), but that good terminal care presupposes the knowing co-operation of the patient. The patient has a right to be consulted about how, when and where terminal care is given, and the patient's participation in decisions about the management of his last days is highly desirable. The conspiracy of silence around the dying patient deceives nobody except perhaps the conspirators themselves. Several studies done with terminal patients have shown that 80–90per cent patients in units where the policy is not to tell patients nevertheless do know that they are dying.[3] Patients pick up this information from various sources: by comparing their symptoms and treatment with other patients, by what they learn indirectly from conversation with other patients and hospital staff (including dinner ladies and porters), by observation of their own deteriorating condition and what their own bodies tell them, and by what they infer from the non-verbal communication of nurses and medical staff (hushed voices, telling looks, silent passing of the bed, over-solicitous care etc). The available evidence suggests that most patients are glad to be told the truth—even if only to put an end to the dreadful uncertainty—and while they may not want to discuss it, most patients do not 'give up', 'turn their faces to the wall', 'go to pieces', provided they are given adequate emotional support and time to come to terms with it.

Similar dilemmas arise for the nurse midwife dealing with the mother who has a stillborn baby. How, when and where does she tell the mother that her baby is dead? Should she tell the father first; Should she let the couple see the baby? How does she cope as a nurse with her own feelings of failure and the need to offer nursing care to the mother afterwards?

In this case the patient not only has a right to know, but is bound to know sooner or later. The grief cannot be avoided. The question is whether the nurse can cope with being the one who tells, sharing the mother's grief, her own likely sense of failure, and continuing to give support afterwards. The inhibition about sharing the truth in this situation has more to do with the nurse's fear of the *responsibility* she accepts in telling the mother, than any question about the mother's rights. Sharing the truth can be a costly business. Once she accepts the responsibility to tell the mother and share her grief with her (and her husband perhaps), she also has to face the difficult practical decisions, requiring tact and judgement, whether the mother will be most helped by being allowed to cuddle her dead baby or needs to be protected from an experience which may be too painful to bear. As long as the nurse is truthful about caring for the mother's needs first and is not simply wanting to hide her own disappointment at not being able to present the mother with a live baby, then she would do best to be guided in what she does by her own common sense.

Because Mary was only thirteen when she was first admitted for treatment for her leukaemia the staff nurse felt that her parents had the right to decide what she should and should not be told. Because she was a minor the staff nurse felt that her parents could override her right to know. Because she was so young the staff nurse felt initially that her parents were right to protect her from the painful truth, but as Mary grew older and asked more searching questions the staff nurse's attitude changed. Did Mary have any more right to know at fifteen than at thirteen? Are parents or relatives entitled to override the rights of dying patients to know the truth, however young or old they are? Would a husband be entitled to refuse to tell his wife that her baby was stillborn?

Because others besides the medical and nursing staff have responsibilities for and obligations to the patient, their judgement needs to be taken into account in assessing how, when and by whom the truth should be told to the patient, but whether any third party has a right to refuse to let the patient ever be told can be seriously doubted on both practical and moral grounds. It depends who is the primary carer and whether or not the patient wishes to exercise their right to know.

A different but related problem about sharing information or telling the truth concerns the converse situation—where the patient knows the truth and refuses to let the medical or nursing staff tell his wife or family. Here there is no direct sense in which we can say that the relatives have a *right* to know because it is not their death that is at issue, but as people who are intimately involved and likely to be affected by the patient's death the nurse may feel that *justice* and compassion demands that they are told. As in the case of Mary, or where the husband prohibits his wife being told about her stillborn child, so here too the nurse may have to use her common sense. It may help to discuss the matter with the person who is prohibiting the disclosure of information to make them aware of how the interests of others are involved, to help them see what comfort may be gained by sharing the truth and the grief together. For example Mary's parents might have been persuaded to tell Mary themselves (with or without the support of the medical and nursing staff); the husband might be persuaded and assisted to tell his wife about the baby himself; the dying patient might need to be encouraged and assisted to share his anxieties and fears about dying with his wife and family and to set his affairs in order. However, if they still refuse the nurse may be able to gain moral support by discussing it with other staff, but in the end the nurse may have to make her own painful decision whether to tell or not. Here she has to balance her responsibility to her patient against her wider responsibility to the family and other concerned parties.

These dilemmas illustrate how truth-sharing is not only a matter of patients' *rights* and staff *responsibility*, or reciprocal rights and responsibilities, but also how considerations of *justice* come into it too. Justice and compassion may demand that the rights of the patient to prohibit the disclosure of confidential information are compromised in the interests of others. The exchange of information, from which the patient derives the right to have his confidences protected, is ultimately concerned with the care, treatment and well-being of the patient. The doctor or nurse may well have to decide in certain circumstances that the disclosure of information to third parties is necessary in the best interests of the patient and in the interests of better patient care. The sharing of information with the family or the rest of the caring team may well be necessary for the proper care of the patient and support of the family.

The patient cannot be considered in isolation, even in his own house. The interests of family, neighbours, community have to be taken into consideration. In hospital the interests of other patients cannot be ignored and the disclosure of information may be necessary to protect the health and safety of other patients. The right to privacy is not an unconditional right. *Justice* demands that if a patient is to benefit from knowledge acquired by the investigation of other patients, then other patients are entitled to benefit from information gathered during his medical examination and treatment. Other patients stand to benefit indirectly from increased knowledge of the medical and social circumstances. It does not mean that nursing staff have to answer anxious or curious questions from other patients. Other patients do not have a right to know even if they are entitled to benefit from the knowledge shared. Nurses must respect the confidences and protect the privacy of patients—unless the matter is of trivial importance.

While seeking to protect the anonymity of the patient, confidential medical information may however have to be disclosed where others may be put at risk if that information is not known (e.g. where there is evidence of child battering). In such cases considerations of justice may well override the rights of the individual patient or the personal obligations which the nurse may feel to her patient.

Deciding between therapeutic and palliative care

The right to treatment is a fundamental right of all patients regardless of their age or whether they can speak for themselves or not. The least problematic situation is where an independent adult, in full possession of his senses, enters into a contract for treatment with a doctor or the caring team when he becomes their patient. In principle, infants and elderly patients have the same rights and are entitled to the same standards of medical care as anyone else. However the situation is complicated when, by reason of physical or mental illness, the patient is in a very dependent and vulnerable condition and decisions have to be taken about their care and treatment by others. The lucid, independent and ambulant patient can actively claim his right to treatment or vote with his feet in refusing treatment. The confused or unconscious, bed-bound or unconsultable patient is in a different position and depends entirely on others to protect his rights and dignity, to ensure that he gets adequate medical treatment and proper nursing care. The infant born with serious physical or mental defects is in the same position and needs to have his interests safeguarded. Just as special tribunals are set up to oversee the care and management of compulsory psychiatric patients, so the courts have a special responsibility to protect the rights of others who are incompetent to defend themselves because of physical or mental infirmity or because of old age or infancy.

This is not because doctors and nurses cannot be trusted to care for their patients in a responsible fashion, but because they need protection as much as their vulnerable patients do, from criticism and litigation or worse. The unconsultable patient needs an independent advocate to represent his interests where there may be doubt and uncertainty about the right course of treatment and conflict between caring professionals about whether the patients' rights have been protected.

Part of the difficulty centres around the ambiguity of the word 'treatment' when we speak of the 'right to treatment'. Treatment embraces *both* medical interventions *and* nursing care, both therapeutic measures and palliative care. In some contexts the purpose of a surgical operation may be to cure— by repairing injury. removing diseased tissue, or preventing the spread of infection. In other contexts surgery may be purely palliative—to relieve pain or to delay the spread of malignant disease. 'Treatment' means both Cure and Care, and it may in practice be very difficult to separate the one from the other. However, most serious dilemmas in terminal care arise when a situation has become ambiguous, when it is not clear whether further therapeutic measures are justified or whether it is necessary 'to settle for comfort'. Definite decisions may be necessary, and there may be conflict between medical and nursing staff about which type of 'treatment' is appropriate and this may be particularly difficult if the patient or relatives are desperately demanding that everything possible should be done or that all treatment should be stopped.

Consider the following three situations described by nurses:

a) When I was a student midwife a baby with Down's syn-drome and a severe heart defect was born to a 38 year old mother and a 42 year old father. Both parents were unable to accept the baby. The father expressed the wish that the baby should not be resuscitated if a crisis occurred. This hap-pened soon afterwards and a junior member of the medical team initiated resuscitation. The baby died after some weeks.

b) In my second year of nursing, during my second spell of night duty as a charge nurse, Margaret was admitted to our ward. She was 23 years old and recently married. She was suffering from oesophageal varices and the consultant surgeon had used a new technique of portal-caval shunt in an attempt to treat her condition. Margaret's condition de-teriorated after the operation and she was in considerable pain. The surgeon insisted she be kept completely drug-free to rest her liver and the resident doctor consequently refused to sign her up for any painkilling drugs, and in-structed me to give a placebo only (whether intravenous or intramuscular).

Margaret was in considerable pain and had more and more distressing nights. She was a most charming person and the staff were very fond of her. This made it very dif-ficult for us, feeling we could not help. In the mornings the ward sister would come on duty, often very early and would demand to know whether Margaret had been sedated. When I told her that I had not been allowed to give her any sedation she would become very angry with me and would (to my relief) instruct me to give her sedation. Each day the same battle would go on between consultant and resident, ward sister and myself, with the nurses concerned to make Margaret as comfortable as possible and the consultant con-cerned that his operation should be a success. The battle continued until very close to Margaret's death, when the consultant surgeon finally conceded that she should be given adequate sedation.

c) While nursing in Accident and Emergency a child victim

of a road traffic accident, with severe injuries and loss of blood, was brought in by her parents. They were Jehovah's Witnesses and insisted that the child should not be given blood transfusions. The parents were asked to wait while X-rays were taken and other tests made. While these were being done it became apparent that the child would not survive without blood transfusions being given. The child was given the necessary transfusions but the parents were not informed. The child survived.

In a), the case of the Down's syndrome baby with congenital heart defect, there are broadly speaking two schools of thought—those that emphasise the rights of the baby and those that emphasise the responsibilities of the medical team. In principle, the baby has the same right to treatment that any adult has and the law should safeguard its rights as it does other vulnerable individuals. An outside party (e.g. a social worker, as in a recent case) should have the right to appeal to the courts to ensure that the child's rights are protected. All citizens have a moral duty to protect the rights of others, and certain professionals such as social workers and hospital chaplains have a special responsibility to act as advocates in the interests of patients whose rights they feel are being compromised or neglected. The parents do not have a moral right to refuse treatment that their child requires to survive, but they cannot be forced to care for the child either. If we recognise that the child has a right to treatment, then we must also recognise that society has an obligation to provide adequate care and support for the child (and possibly for the parents as well).

In practice the situation is more complicated, because the social provision for the care of severely handicapped children is inadequate, and support for affected families insufficient to prevent severe hardship and distress. Compassion for the parents who quite understandably may feel unable to cope, and for the medical staff who are faced with immediate decisions about care and treatment for the child, may seem to point in the direction of letting nature take its course and allowing the child to die. In reality the medical team and the parents have to try to resolve the situation in the most responsible way. The risks of medical intervention are that the child would still be left severely handicapped for life, and would require pretty constant medical care and attention through life. The parents would almost inevitably have to carry the main burden of caring for the child because of the lack of practical alternatives. (The same problems arise with spina bifida babies.) The painful reality is that the child's right to treatment and the medical team's duty to care have to be worked out in most cases in a social setting where there is inadequate social provision for the care and support of such children and their families. This places unjust pressure on the family to accept responsibilities greater than they can cope with on their own, and on the medical team who may not feel free to do what is in the child's best interests. This illustrates how issues of rights cannot be separated from justice and questions concerning the allocation of resources in society generally. If we feel strongly about the rights of defective newborns to adequate care and treatment, we also have to be willing to campaign for a more just society and adequate services for all, including the most vulnerable

Clinical decisions in such cases are not unambiguous. Past experience may show that there is little hope for such cases or that in some cases medical or surgical intervention can be successful in ensuring survival and a reasonable quality of life. However medical evidence will not be enough to resolve the moral dilemma, and quality of life arguments are very subjective. (Who is to say that a painful handicapped life is worse than no life at all?) The infant certainly has a right to treatment but it does not follow that that means that *everything* possible has to be tried, including the most expensive, untried or dangerous treatments. Treatment, as we have said, may mean direct interventions which aim to cure, or it may mean provision of nursing care and symptom control. Deciding which is appropriate in such a case may be difficult and morally ambiguous. It may be tempting to simply 'treat' the parents' distress or the medical team's anxiety by removing the object that is causing it, but that would not represent the kind of courageous initiative which the situation demands—a courage to act in spite of the practical uncertainty and moral ambiguity and accept the consequences.

The distinction drawn by moral theologians between 'ordinary' and 'extraordinary' means—when they say that medical staff are obliged to offer the child the 'ordinary' means of assistance, but not obliged to employ 'extraordinary' means in the attempt to save its life—does not solve the moral dilemma in such cases, but points to the need for decisions based on common sense and regard for the circumstances and needs of all parties with a responsibility to care. 'Leaving nature to take its course' seldom means doing nothing more for the affected infant. It may mean continuing to give fluids (and possibly food or drugs to suppress hunger), keeping the infant comfortable and pain-free. Or it may mean not intervening actively to give antibiotics, or to perform surgery with a poor record of success, and not resuscitating the infant if it suffers cardiac arrest. In the case we are considering, the houseman acted decisively to resuscitate the child but she died anyway. His action was a perfectly understandable one. It was one possible response to a distressing situation, one possible attempt to resolve a painful dilemma. It is an action which has its own possible medical and moral justification. (The child did after all survive for a few extra days.) However it might have been no less morally courageous, and possibly more difficult in the face of the pressure 'to do something', to have left the child to die. Such situations are called dilemmas because there is no way you can know unambiguously what is right to do in the circumstances.[4]

Not taking any action to resuscitate a patient who has suffered cardiac arrest or choked, is sometimes referred to as *passive euthanasia* (in contrast to *active euthanasia* when someone directly assists a patient to die). Some moral philosophers argue that there is an important distinction between active killing and letting die, in terms of the different intentions of the agent, and therefore that while active euthanasia is not morally acceptable, in some circumstances passive euthanasia may be. Other philosophers argue that in terms of consequences (the death of the patient) there is really no difference between them. There are complex arguments on both sides but the medical and nursing professions have long accepted that there is a common-sense distinction between actively killing a patient (with or without his consent) and taking no action to save their life when they are dying.

However, this common-sense distinction, as well as the distinction between 'ordinary' and 'extraordinary' means, is put under strain when we consider what has been made possible by the development of modern drugs, anaesthetics and life support machines. To some extent the boundaries between 'ordinary' and 'extraordinary' are changing all the the time and that does not make these decisions any easier. The presence or absence of sophisticated resuscitative equipment can make all the difference to how a case is viewed. Is actively switching off a life-support system to a brain-dead patient (being kept 'alive' for transplant purposes) active or passive euthanasia? Or neither? With more precise medical and legal criteria for defining death this particular dilemma may be removed, but with live patients who are dying the problems remain.

In case b), the conflict between the nurses and the doctors over the level of pain-control to be given to Margaret, we encounter a common problem in doctor/nurse relationships in terminal care. The problem relates partly to the different functions of the nurse and the doctor and their perceived roles in relation to the severely ill patient. However it also tends to arise in the pre-terminal stage when it is as yet unclear whether the patient is dying or her life may be saved. While there is hope curative measures are appropriate even to the point of refusing sedation if it may jeopardise a cure. Once the situation is recognised to be hopeless, then appropriate palliative care should be given. Deciding when it is appropriate to switch from theraputic measures to palliative treatment may be very difficult and fraught with uncertainty. The anxiety of the doctor not to be found wanting drives him to do all he can, while the anxiety of the nursing staff at having to cope with the distress of the patient may drive them to demand that they should 'settle for comfort'. The doctor's experience that patients (especially young patients) may sometimes be 'snatched from the jaws of Death' has to be balanced against the experience of nurses when patients have 'turned the corner never to return'. Decisions about the type of management appropriate may have to be taken under pressure from rebellious nurses, or by the doctor insisting on his medical authority, but they do have to be taken.

A common dilemma in such circumstances relates to the use of powerful pain-controlling drugs such as diamorphine which nevertheless have dangerous side-effects (e.g. suppressing respiratory function) which may hasten the patient's death or make them more susceptible to infections which may kill them. Some nurses object to giving diamorphine to dying patients even if they are in great pain because they regard this as a form of euthanasia. Even more are afraid of being the one who administers the last injection and may appear to be responsible for the death of the patient. Clearly a nurse has a right to refuse to do something which violates her conscience, but she may need help to understand that the patient has a right to treatment in such a situation even if it shortens his or her life. Some moral theologians have used the 'argument from double effect' to provide a common-sense moral justification for the use of measures which have both a desirable effect, such as relieving severe pain, and the undesirable effect of possibly shortening the patient's life. If the primary intention is to relieve pain (and not to kill the patient) then the secondary effect though foreseen, is not one for which one is responsible in the same way as if one had deliberately set out to kill the patient. This argument, though not solving the dilemma, may help some people to cope with the painful responsibility involved.

Better knowledge of pain-control, and experience gained in terminal care units, has shown that proper use of diamorphine and other drugs can not only greatly improve the quality of life of the patient who is dying, but may actually give them the strength and determination to live longer.

Case c), the case of the child of Jehovah's Witness parents, raises in an acute form the question of whether children have the same rights as adults and if so how they are to be protected. In the circumstances the medical and nursing staff colluded in deceiving the parents so as to ensure that the child was given the necessary life-saving blood transfusions. They clearly felt that the parents did not have the moral right to refuse the child treatment it required for survival. They might have applied to a judge and had the child made a Ward of Court and this might have been a more proper procedure to adopt to protect themselves from litigation. However, problems remain. Given the beliefs held by Jehovah's Witnesses there was a risk that the parents would subsequently reject the child and if they did, a question as to whether society would be willing and able to provide the child with adequate alternative care.

Where such a clash of values between parents and professionals takes place, the interpretation of rights and responsibilities becomes a matter of disagreement. The medical and nursing staff in such a situation should ideally make their own moral and legal viewpoint clear to the parents, and attempt to persuade them to accept the necessity for treatment while trying to accomodate their wishes where possible by the use of other measures. However, if no other course is open to them, they may have to act despite the parents' wishes, and have a right to expect that the courts and society would give them and the child the necessary support.

NOTES AND REFERENCES

1. Masters R D 1975 Is contract an adequate basis for medical care? and May W F 1975 Code, covenant, contract or philanthropy. Hastings Centre Report 5 (December): 24–38
2. Thompson I E 1975 Dilemmas of dying. University Press, Edinburgh, ch 5
3. Abrams R D 1966 The patient with cancer, his changing pattern of communication. New England Journal of Medicine 274: 317–322
   Benoliel J Q 1970 Talking to patients about death. Nursing Forum 9(3)
   Hinton J 1972 Dying. Penguin Books, Harmondsworth, ch 8
   Hinton J 1979 Comparison of places and policies for terminal care. Lancet Jan 6
   Parkes C M 1966 The patient's right to know the truth. Proceedings of the Royal Society of Medicine 66: 536
   In a recent unpublished study conducted by staff of St Columba's Hospice, Edinburgh, 85–90% of patients interviewed before admission knew that they had a terminal illness.
4. Stinson R, Stinson P 1981 On the death of a baby. Journal of Medical Ethics 7(1): 5–18
5. Harris J 1981 Ethical problems in the management of some severely handicapped children. Journal of Medical Ethics 7(3): 117–124

5

Moral dilemmas in nursing groups of patients

Responsibility for individuals and responsibility for groups of patients

In the previous chapter we discussed two classes of moral dilemma in direct nurse/patient encounters; these centred on dilemmas of truth-telling and confidentiality on the one hand and dilemmas of deciding between therapeutic and palliative treatment on the other. While these could not be discussed entirely without regard to the rights of other patients and relatives, the second two groups of moral dilemmas cannot be discussed without taking account of the rights of other patients or the good of society. These are dilemmas which relate to

a) setting limits to the control and direction of patients

b) balancing the rights of patients and the interests of third parties.

It may be useful in this connection to distinguish a little more clearly between four different, but related senses of responsibility:

Responsibility *for* one's own actions (Personal Responsibility)

Responsibility *for* the care of someone else (Fiduciary Responsibility)

Responsibility *to* higher authority (Professional Accountability)

Responsibility *to* wider society (Civic Duty)

Personal responsibility. One is ordinarily held responsible for one's own actions and praised or blamed for them, provided one knows what one is doing, has acted freely and voluntarily and provided one can distinguish between right and wrong. This sense of responsibility applies to all one's actions and is the most basic sense involved when one is being tried for negligence by a court or investigating inquiry. Here excusing conditions which may be taken into account in determining the degree of guilt involved are: ignorance, stress of circumstances, inexperience in making moral decisions of the kind in question.

Fiduciary responsibility. When someone is entrusted to your care (e.g. a child, an unconscious or mentally disordered patient), or when a patient voluntarily entrusts his life into your hands, you acquire what is called fiduciary responsibility (from the Latin *fiducia*, meaning trust). Thus having responsibility for the care and treatment of patients, or decisions about their individual and collective well-being, is a matter of fiduciary responsibility, and the power or authority of the nurse to do these things derives from the trust which the patient and society places in her.

Professional Accountability. Because of the responsibility vested in the nurse by patients and society, and underwritten by the professional nursing associations and the General Nursing Council, the nurse has an obligation or duty to give account of her actions to her peers, her superiors, to the GNC, and to society through the courts, if necessary. This duty of public accountability follows from the responsibilities entrusted to her as a professional. Many nurses will feel directly accountable to patients and to relatives as well, but this can be to confuse their duty to care for these people in the widest sense (including respecting their right to know) with accountability in the strict sense which refers only to one's profession and to higher authority. In some cases it will not be helpful (or wise) for the nurse to give all the reasons for her actions to patients and relatives—at least not until demanded to do so by an enquiry. From the daily Kardex meeting and meetings of the medical care team, through to enquiries by the GMC and the courts, the professional is obliged to give account of himself in virtue of the trust vested in him.

Civic duty. The nurse as a professional is a member of a public body with corporate responsibilities. As professional member of the National Health Service staff the nurse has responsibility for maintaining the general standards of nursing care. As members of a profession committed to the care of patients nurses have responsibilities to influence health policy and the allocation of resources. Nurses are public officers, even public servants, with both civic and political duties. They have individual civic responsibility to society to draw attention to specific examples of incompetence or negligence or where standards of care have become unacceptable. They have public or political responsibility to act corporately, through nursing unions or associations, to try to bring about changes in practice, improved standards of care, more appropriate allocation of resources, more relevant health policies—for the benefit of patients as a whole.

When nurses are compelled to consider their responsibility for individual patients against the background of their responsibilities for groups of patients, conflicts may arise between these different responsibilities which the nurse carries as a professional. The authority vested in her, to serve the best interests of her patients, may contrast with the actual or relative lack of power which she has—depending on her relationships with other staff, her position in the nursing hierarchy, what she is entitled to do by law and what she is or is not allowed to do by her union or professional associations. Some of these dilemmas of responsibility and authority are among those to which we now turn.

Setting limits to the control and direction of patients

The management of patients is a complex art—ranging from subtle persuasion to the use of force to subdue violent patients. What gives the nurse the authority to control other people in this way?

In psychiatric wards, in accident and emergency departments and in working with the mentally handicapped, nurses often encounter violent patients who have to be restrained by physical means, by the use of drugs or by invoking the law. In such cases it may appear that the nursing staff are justified in using force to control patients simply in order to defend themselves and to defend other patients and staff. They may also be acting to protect the patient from injury, self-mutilation or suicide, or, less dramatically, acting to protect their own best interests.[1]

The fact is that the nurse is not only responsible for the individual patient and his needs, nor solely concerned with his rights. The nurse also has to protect the interests of other patients and, as a public officer who is accountable to society at large, has to consider the public good. The rights of individual patients may have to be restricted where the rights of other people are put at risk. In addition, the nurse has a responsibility to protect the interests of the patient who is incapable of understanding what his own best interests are—e.g. if he is mentally ill, intoxicated or mentally handicapped. The nurse has to decide what is in the best interests of the patient and good patient care. The nurse is entrusted with this responsibility (sometimes called fiduciary responsibility) and must be guided in the decisions she makes by her training and experience, professional code and personal conscience.[1]

Concern with the 'common good' and the 'best interests' of the patient means that the nurse exercises both clinical and moral responsibilities towards her patients. These are determined not only by consideration of their rights and respect for their freedom, but also by consideration of the wider health needs of the individual and the community. 'Management' of patients (including those who co-operate fully in treatment) can involve various degrees of control, ranging from physical restraint or legal measures, to behavioural modification, health education and simply directive managerial communication. Skill in nursing means, in part at least, learning to control people in the nicest possible way.

Moral responsibility and personal freedom

Consider the following problem encountered by a psychiatric nurse:

> On our ward we recently had a 70 year old woman who was described as an alcoholic and had taken several overdoses over a period of two years. The staff feared that if she was discharged she would return home to her alcoholic husband

and sooner or later would be found dead. However when she was sober she appeared completely rational and demanded to be allowed home. Her compulsory detention in hospital on the grounds that she might commit suicide seemed to me a flagrant violation of her freedom when there did not appear to be adequate evidence that she was mentally ill.

The same nurse went on to ask whether a nurse has a duty to prevent someone from committing suicide if they want to do so.

As long as the person is a patient in their care the law requires the nurse to protect them from harm and that includes self-inflicted harm. In fact a nurse can be charged with negligence if a patient succeeds in killing themselves. The nurse has this legal duty towards patients in her care in spite of the fact that it is no longer illegal for someone to attempt suicide. The law assumes that the instinct for self-preservation is natural in man and that acts of self-destruction indicate that 'the balance of a person's mind has been disturbed'. As mentally unbalanced they are not prosecuted but by the same token health professionals are expected to care for them and protect them from themselves. Most religious and virtually all human societies disapprove of suicide and therefore most nurses feel a *moral* obligation to prevent people from killing themselves as well. The fact that the law allows people the licence or liberty to attempt suicide without prosecution does not mean that the law or morality recognises that persons have a *right* to kill themselves. We could only properly speak of a 'right to commit suicide' if other people had a corresponding responsibility to assist them to do so.

In the case just mentioned the ambiguity arises because of the uncertainty about the elderly woman's mental state. Was the woman capable of making rational decisions about her life? The action of the hospital in protecting her might appear paternalistic and restrictive of the woman's liberty, but it could be said to be a natural extension of her right to treatment and the contract of the staff to care for her (as well as to offer her such therapy as might be appropriate). Here the nurse has to exercise fiduciary responsibility on behalf of the patient and that may involve restricting her movements.

The least generous construction which could be placed on the action of the hospital is that the staff were acting less to protect the old lady than to protect themselves against the charge of negligence and the guilt which might result if the patient succeeded in killing herself. The fact is that no matter what precautions are taken some patients do succeed in committing suicide and that does cause great distress to the staff responsible for their care. Nevertheless, defensive action and conservative measures, though they may be somewhat repressive at times, are not morally unjustifiable. On the contrary, staff are entitled to protect themselves and their professional reputations. The courage to take the risk of discharging a potentially suicidal patient may show admirable regard for their autonomy but can always be attacked as irresponsibility. Achieving a balance between caring for and protecting patients and respecting their freedom, between defensive medicine and attempted rehabilitation, is always difficult, a matter of risk and often complicated by the risk of legal action.

Behaviour modification

Another type of control which raises ethical problems is the use of rewards and punishments to reinforce behaviour modification in long-term psychiatric patients. For example, money or cigarettes may be given as rewards to encourage better self-care among severely institutionalised patients—e.g. for washing, shaving, dressing, bed-making, care of living area, and sanctions may be applied e.g. by the removal of privileges such as access to television, opportunities for exercise or recreation. Is it ethically justifiable to extend the definition of treatment to include the re-training and rehabilitation of patients by these means?

Health-care staff, trained to standards of cleanliness, order and tidiness, may find the slovenliness of some patients intolerable. (As community nurses may find offensive the behaviour of elderly people with what has been called the 'Diogenes syndrome'.) It is easy to rationalise the use of re-training measures for such patients on the grounds that it is necessary for reasons of hygiene, to avoid fire hazards and to protect other patients' interests. Re-training patients to care for themselves and their environment may also ease the burden on the nursing staff and make the institutional management of such individuals easier and more pleasant. Each of these kinds of reason may carry some weight in justifying the use of behaviour modification techniques, but, unless they are balanced by respect for the patient's rights and autonomy, could lead to abuse.

The use of aversion therapy in the treatment of some phobias and in assisting people to give up smoking, the abuse of drugs, or alcohol, can be justified reasonably easily in practice because the patient generally wants help to overcome the phobia or dependence on addictive substances and can, as a rule, be consulted about treatment and give their informed and voluntary consent.

These cases are reasonably straightforward when the patient is competent to give consent. The case is much more complicated when the patient is mentally handicapped, mentally ill, senile or suffering the consequences of long-term institutionalisation. Here there may be serious doubts whether consent can be either informed or voluntary in any adequate sense. It becomes a matter of fiduciary responsibility on the part of the health care staff. They have to fall back on other kinds of justification: arguments that such measures are ultimately in the best interests of the patient, or that the re-training is necessary to protect the rights (health and safety) of others, or that the staff cannot be obliged to work in intolerable conditions.[2]

The argument that it is in the *best interests* of the patient is acceptable if and only if it is informed by a proper respect for the dignity of individual patients, by a concern to rehabilitate them or at least to improve the general standards of patient care. Respect for the dignity of persons will obviously set limits to the degree or forms of coercion which are employed and even the use of cigarettes as inducements may be ruled out on the grounds that they may damage the health of patients. There is always a risk that the assumption of fiduciary responsibility may lead to paternalism and even the abuse of patients if it is not limited by respect for persons. The argument that it is necessary to *protect the rights of others* has more force in some circumstances, provided there is real evidence of risk. Studies of the extent of fire risk among mildly demented elderly people, for example, have shown that the risk is much less than it is imagined to be by neighbours and anxious professionals and that the use of alternative forms of heating can sometimes circumvent the need for institutionalisation.[3] It is far too easy for health professionals to rationalise their prejudices against people with a different lifestyle or standards of cleanliness, and to impose a regimen on patients for their own convenience rather than the real benefit of patients. If this is recognised, then there may well be reason to use behaviour modification techniques for the rehabilitation of those whose standards of self-care have deteriorated with illness or institutionalisation. The rights of staff to decent working conditions are important but not so important as to justify coercion of patients to conform to staff demands, when perhaps collective action may be necessary by nurses to ensure better staffing levels, modernisation of equipment and the provision of adequate resources.

Health education

Health Education itself, insofar as it seeks to change people's attitudes and behaviour, raises ethical questions as well: are nurses entitled to tell people that they should stop smoking, should not drink so much, or that they should go on diet? Or, more controversially, are they morally justified in advising people to practice contraception or to seek sterilization? If so how directive should they be? Should they just give people the facts and leave them to decide for themselves? Should they actively try to change people's attitudes and life-style? Should they be campaigning for legislation to control advertising of alcohol and tobacco? Should they support compulsory seat-belt legislation, drunk driving laws or compulsory fluoridation? Should they be involved directly in community development in areas of high unemployment and social deprivation?[4]

Health education, if it is to be relevant, must be related to the patterns of morbidity and mortality in society. In the past the infectious diseases and diseases associated with poverty were responsible for very high infant mortality rates and the deaths of young people. These have been largely controlled by general improvements in the standard of living (better housing and diet), public health measures (better sewerage disposal, cleaner water supplies), and by medical measures (immunisation and the development of effective drugs). Today, in the developed countries, the pattern of morbidity and mortality is quite different. Infant mortality rates have been dramatically reduced and most dying is done by the elderly. There has been a vast increase in the proportion of the population over the age of fifty and most illness in this group is lifestyle-related. Apart from accidental and violent deaths (a small proportion) the vast majority of deaths and morbidity in the population are associated with smoking, alcohol abuse, inappropriate diet and lack of exercise. While poverty and its associated conditions of multiple deprivation are important factors, the epidemic of chronic and disabling diseases of middle and later life is clearly lifestyle-related. If smoking, alcohol abuse and poor diet are to be eliminated as major causes of disease in society, then people's attitudes and values, their lifestyle, has to be changed.

Obviously the major ethical justification for health education is the same as that which was invoked to justify compulsory immunisation, notification of infectious diseases, and compulsory public health measures: namely, an appeal to the *common good*—the protection of the rights (to health and safety) of the majority, even if it meant restricting the rights of some individuals and dissenting minorities. (The issues of compulsory seat-belt legislation or fluoridation raise similar questions today.) The fact is however that legal and fiscal measures cannot be forced on a community entirely without their consent, even in a totalitarian state. Public opinion has to be informed and persuaded, a consensus created—and that is a task of health education. If health education is not to give offence it has to respect the rights and autonomy of individuals, their right to decide on their own values and lifestyle. People cannot be forced to take responsibility for their health. They may be persuaded to do so, given inducements to do so or subject to various forms of sanctions if they do not do so. So if health education is to be effective, it may be necessary for a wide variety of health education measures to be used. It will not be sufficient just to give people the facts and leave them to make up their own minds when millions of pounds are spent annually on advertising alcohol and tobacco. It will not be sufficient to promote the value of positive health through the education of individuals—both schoolchildren and adults—when these alternative attitudes and values are contradicted by the social circumstances in which they live. It will not be sufficient to try to influence health behaviour through taxation and legal measures when huge vested interests are at stake in the tobacco, alcohol and food industries. Advertising may need to be controlled, funds may have to be allocated for community development and the combatting of social deprivation and poverty, state subsidies and tax incentives may need to be given to companies to diversify and phase out the increasing production of things damaging to our health.

Health professionals have a fundamental responsibility to be health educators, insofar as their training as doctors and nurses or paramedicals must commit them to the promotion of health, and not merely the treatment of disease. The National Health Service is not and never has been intended to be purely a National Disease Service. Health professionals have a responsibility for the *health* of their patients. The health professional therefore has a special responsibility to act as a role model. The nurse who is a heavy smoker or abuses alcohol cannot expect her advice to be taken seriously. Her credibility as a health professional is called in question. This does not mean that all nurses have to be angels, but their example in taking responsibility for their own health is important. The high cigarette consumption among nurses as a profession may have many explanations, including the alternating periods of stress and boredom which characterises their work. However, the example of doctors in giving up smoking has not only had a dramatic effect on the incidence of heart disease and lung cancer in their ranks, but has obviously impressed their patients, who have given up smoking in large numbers.

Health professionals, as a body of people with public responsibility for maintaining the health services, cannot simply rest content with passively implementing health policies decided by other people. As those who see the casualties on the wards and in the community every day, they have a responsibility to try to use their political influence actively to shape health policies. Through their professional associations and unions nurses have the power to influence public opinion to achieve by political, legislative and fiscal means what cannot be achieved by individual counselling. However, respect for the rights of individuals can and must be maintained when pressure is being exerted on individuals and nations to change their lifestyle. The ultimate justification for health education is that the rights of patients demand it—especially the right to know and the right to treatment.

Communication

Communication with patients is not only important as a means of discovering or conveying information, and as a means of expressing sympathy, encouragement and personal interest, but it is also the single most important way of securing patient co-operation and compliance. In a word, communication plays a vital role in the *management and control of patients*.[5, 6]

It has become fashionable to talk about the importance of communication in medicine and nursing, and to explain the failures in doctor/patient and nurse/patient relationships as due to poor communication. This is misleading if it means that in general doctors and nurses are poor communicators. In fact they are highly skilled at certain kinds of communication and less good at others. Experienced doctors and nurses are highly skilled at certain forms of directive managerial communication—using language and the selective disclosure of information as a means of securing patient compliance and as a means of controlling them. However they may be much less skilled than their junior colleagues at communicating with patients as persons, understanding their personal needs, responding to their different levels of comprehension of information. Training and the demands of institutional life and the need to 'manage' large numbers of patients may make them less sensitive with the passage of time to the way manipulative communication can offend patients and create mistrust. (Patients often remark that they learn more from porters and cleaners than from medical and nursing staff, and these hospital staff have an important role to play in communication with patients.)

Communication between nurses and patients can raise two kinds of ethical problems: first when communication fails to express respect for the patient as a person; and second when the patient's right to know is ignored. The first kind of problem arises when hospital staff literally talk over the heads of their patients or, more seriously, fail to respect their confidences. The power-relationship between patient and professional is an unequal one and communication can be used in such a way that its primary purpose is to control the patient rather than to relate to him as a person. The sick or injured patient is often anxious and distressed because he does not understand what is happening to him or why it is happening. He is vulnerable and dependent and needs the help of the professional to understand. He does not only need the reassurance which the expert can give him, but he needs information—the benefit of the expert's knowledge. The medical and nursing staff are in a controlling position—offering care and treatment, possessing expert knowledge and having specific information about the needs, condition, treatment and likely prognosis of the patient. They have a responsibility to share their knowledge and this specific information about the patient with him, and to share it in the most caring way. The disclosure of information can be used merely as a means of controlling patients or as an expression of real care for their needs. Because the patient is generally 'sick, ignorant and horizontal' while the staff are 'well, knowledgeable and vertical', they have natural advantages which must not be abused.

Balancing the rights of patients with the interests of third parties

In general, doctors and nurses are trained to view their moral responsibilities in *personal* terms with specific reference to the one-to-one relationship between doctor and patient, or nurse and patient in the clinical situation. In practice doctors and nurses usually have obligations to several other patients at the same time and therefore have to consider their interests as well. Because each nurse has only one pair of hands and cannot be in two places at once she has to make decisions about whom to give priority and how to do the best for all her patients. These more *universal* considerations of justice and the common good may often suggest different responses to her than if she only had one patient to care for. The same could be said for doctors. The demands of teaching, administration, research and public health all introduce more universal obligations which have to be balanced against the rights of patients in the one-to-one clinical relationship.

Health professionals often feel most comfortable at the level of ethical decisions of a personal kind relating to individual patients and their health needs. The doctor's expertise and clinical judgement relate most appropriately to the treatment of individual patients and decisions about their management, and a personal ethic based on care is most appropriate to such situations. The doctor may well feel that his expertise (unless he is an epidemiologist and trained administrator) is less appropriate to decisions about the general allocation of man-power and resources. Nurses on the other hand, while sharing the same personalist ethic, may have more experience in decisions about management of large groups of patients and feel less uneasy about making decisions based on the general good. The conflict between these different kinds of values, personalist and universal, come out most clearly where the rights of individual patients have to be balanced against the interests of third parties. The following situations may serve to illustrate some of the problems and dilemmas: decisions about termination of pregnancy, therapeutic and non-therapeutic medical research, the use of patients as teaching material, and decisions about the allocation of resources.

Termination of pregnancy

It may seem strange to discuss abortion under the heading of personal and universal interests, but it may be useful to do so because it illustrates clearly that a personalist ethic based on the duty to care is not sufficient to deal with a situation where a conflict arises between the rights of two patients—particularly when one is inside the other!

Consider the following situation described by a student mid-wife:

During my training I was working in a gynaecological ward where some of the women were in hospital for termination of pregnancy. One of the patients was a married woman who already had three children. Part of the reason why she wanted a termination was that the child she was carrying was not her husband's. She was around 16 weeks pregnant and the method used for termination was hypertonic saline.

This lady was extremely upset on admission to the ward, and very aware and sensitive about the situation which had forced her to this decision. She was very fond of her three children and her husband and could not think what had made her sleep with this other man.

The attitude to the patient of several of the senior nursing staff could only be described as hostile. This amazed me as they were usually fairly sympathetic and supportive to the other patients who were admitted for termination. A lot of the hostility appeared to be due to the fact that the patient was an older woman and, in their eyes, should have known better. Their attitude which they made fairly plain to the patient only served to heighten her feeling of guilt and shame.

As a student nurse I was appalled at this attitude, as I believe vulnerable patients depend on nurses to be supportive and understanding.

In this case the student midwife did not appear to disapprove of abortion, nor did the senior nurses, but they disagreed in their attitudes to the unfortunate woman with her illegitimate child and what appeared to be her reasons for seeking termination of her pregnancy. The student midwife bases her judgement solely upon her response to the individual patient, identifying with her personal and moral predicament. The senior nurses, on her account, consider those reasons inadequate to seek a mid-term abortion. We may speculate that they consider the woman and her husband have a responsibility to seek other solutions rather than abortion to solve their interpersonal problems. The point which this case illustrates is the tension between approaches based on regard for the mother alone and an approach which takes account of the interests of the other parties involved.

The issue of abortion is fiercely debated by the pro-life (anti-abortion) groups and those (pro-abortion) groups that seek to uphold the woman's right to choose. The pro-lifers emphasise the rights of the unborn child and the pro-abortionists the rights of the pregnant woman.

Arguments rage about whether the foetus has rights and if so at what stage it acquires them—at conception, at viability, at birth. Is a foetus a person in the legal and moral sense? Why does the law allow an unborn child the right to inherit property and the child the right to sue for injury or damage suffered before birth, but allow the foetus to be destroyed or killed by abortion? Arguments rage about the rights of women—the right to control their own fertility, to choose whether or not to continue a pregnancy, the right to abortion on demand.

What are the limits of individual rights when other life is at stake? Why does the law permit abortions to be performed but not give women an automatic right to termination of pregnancy?

Clearly the issue of rights is complicated. The fact is that the 1967 UK Abortion Act is merely an enabling act. In terms of the Act it is no longer illegal to procure an abortion or to assist in terminating a pregnancy. The parties involved are no longer liable to prosecution provided the conditions of the Act are met: that the continuation of the pregnancy would put at risk the physical or mental health of the patient and that the termination is approved by two doctors. This does not mean that the Act creates a 'right to abortion', but it allows the liberty to terminate a pregnancy. It would only be said to have created a 'right to abortion' if doctors and nurses were obliged to assist with terminations. In theory at least, the conscience clause allows dissenting doctors and nurses to refuse to do so in some areas, just as it may be difficult in other areas for women to get assistance in terminating a pregnancy. Even if the law did recognise a right to abortion on demand it could not be an unconditional right without violating the rights of those health professionals who conscientiously object to abortion.

The question of the rights of the foetus is even more complicated. Disagreements about the moral and legal status of foetuses, that is whether they are persons and have rights, leave considerable ambiguity. To defend their rights, like the rights of the mentally handicapped or the demented elderly, we have to invoke more universal considerations of justice, compassion and humanity. A conception of personal rights based on respect for persons is not adequate when the status of individuals as persons is in doubt.

A definition of who is to qualify for membership of the moral community, of the human family, requires that we extend for reasons of justice and beneficience the rights which are proper to adults of sound mind, to children, to those who are dying or suffering degeneration of their faculties as well as to the unborn. However no-one's rights are absolute and unconditional, and painful dilemmas may arise when there is a conflict of rights and two lives are at stake.

The painful position of the nurse or doctor is related to the fact that on the one hand their immediate responsibility is to the person who presents for treatment or help—in this case the mother—and on the other hand the principle of benefi- cience which is fundamental to the codes of medical and nurs- ing practice—to do no harm, to preserve life, to protect the weak and to act as an advocate for those in their care—gives them a special responsibility to care for vulnerable foetal life. Where the interests of mother and foetus conflict, impossible dilemmas arise. These are reflected in fundamental disagree- ments about the kind of balance of rights involved and even in the terminology to be used to describe the contents of the pregnant woman's womb. The 'pro-life' group (like the Society for the Protection of the Unborn Child) speak of the 'unborn child' and thereby seek to emphasise their belief that the rights of the foetus are equal to or greater than the mother's. The use of terms like 'foetus' or 'conceptus' by the 'pro-abortion' lobby expresses their conviction that the rights of the mother are paramount and that the foetus has lesser rights or that it has no rights at all. The debate between these two camps, though polarised and often acrimonious, may be important as a means of highlighting areas in our moral thinking where we have not yet reached a clear moral consensus, in particular about the rights of women and the rights of foetal life.

It has been remarked that when people have recourse to the language of 'rights', when people start demanding the right to work, the right to strike or the right to abortion on demand, they are doing three things: first, they are drawing attention to an area of felt injustice; second, they are defining prescrip- tively what they think ought to be their rights; and third, they are trying to persuade others to agree with them and support the campaign to have their rights recognised.

In this case, two opposing ideological groups are concerned with two different areas of felt or feared injustice. The 'pro- abortion' lobby are mainly concerned about the injustice suf- fered by women in a society where they do not in reality enjoy equal rights with men and in practice suffer sexual exploitation in many forms. The right to control their own fertility, includ- ing the right to terminate a pregnancy, is seen as fundamental to resisting this injustice and exploitation and achieving greater equality with men. (The de-medicalisation of contraception may also be a necessary means to achieve this end.) The 'pro- life' lobby fear the injustice that may be suffered by dependent and vulnerable unborn children if they are relegated to the status of mere 'foetuses' or 'conceptuses' without personal rights. The fear is that this will lead to lack of sensitivity to vulnerable life in other forms and disregard for the rights of defective newborns, the severely handicapped or demented elderly. Infanticide and selective euthanasia of incompetents are feared as consequences of any lessening of vigilance in the protection of the legal and moral rights of all human life.

While these ideological disputes may serve to highlight the human rights issues which are at stake, and may eventually lead to clarification of agreed principles for a new social consensus, they do not necessarily help decide practical dilemmas in specific cases. It may be necessary to recognise that in the sometimes tragic complexity of life no ideal solution is possible. It may not be possible to resolve the dilemma at a theoretical level, but some practical decision has to be taken and the only possible way out may be to choose the lesser of two evils. However, specific decisions like this should not be generalised into universal solutions. Each case should be considered on its own terms in the light of experience and general moral principles.

In general, few would say that abortion is desirable for its own sake. Most would agree that if all pregnancies were the result of loving and responsible planning by the partners, if ideal forms of contraception were freely available, and if society was not unwilling for young people to be properly informed about sex and contraception, then the problem of unwanted pregnancies and the demand for abortion would not arise—except in cases where it is indicated for therapeutic reasons. However these ideal conditions do not exist and the number of pregnancies among unmarried teenagers is increasing at an alarming rate (currently some 7 000 per annum in Scotland alone) and with it the demand for terminations.

Some people believe it is never justifiable to terminate a pregnancy, others that it is justifiable in certain circumstances, as the lesser of two evils (for example, where the life of the mother is in danger or for other grave reasons). Those who advocate more liberal abortion policies do not generally agree that abortion should be allowed for trivial reasons, and even those who argue for the woman's right to choose abortion on demand must recognise that no rights, not even women's rights, can be absolute or unconditional. However the 'problem of abortion' cannot be solved on the basis of arguments based on human rights alone. At a theoretical level, considerations of justice for all parties involved and the duty to care have to be taken into account. At a practical level, the consequences of terminating or not terminating a particular pregnancy have to be carefully considered in the light of the cost in human suffering or benefit for the parties involved. Further, the adoption of a pro-abortion policy or an anti-abortion policy is not enough to protect women's rights or the rights of foetal life unless there is a commitment to the education of society about responsible and caring relationships and changes in the status and rights of women.

Therapeutic and non-therapeutic medical research

Medical science can only advance through properly controlled scientific research. The controls required are both scientific and ethical. Research which is not conducted according to proper scientific procedure is valueless, and research which is not conducted with proper respect for the rights of patients may become inhuman.

In order to be *scientific*, medical research must be based on proper scientific knowledge, prior laboratory and animal experiments and proper research design, and be conducted by properly qualified research staff.

In order to be *ethical* medical research must be based on prior assessment of risks and benefits of the research procedures (and would not be justified when the risks outweigh the benefits). Further it would have to be based on the full informed and voluntary consent of the patient to his participation in the research project, or, where the patient is not competent to give consent, special safefugards must be established to protect the patient's rights (e.g. proxy consent or tribunals to monitor the research in the patient's interest).[7]

Medical research may be therapeutic or non-therapeutic. It is called therapeutic if it is directly related to the patient's complaint and if they stand to benefit directly from the drugs or procedures which are used. Non-therapeutic medical research is research where patients participate in general investigations which are aimed at improving knowledge of body chemistry or body function and may have no direct therapeutic purpose or relevance. In practice the distinction is not so clear-cut, for patients may stand to benefit in the long-run from even the most academic studies of the composition of the blood or the biochemistry of the brain, for example, and in randomised control trials using placebos some patients may receive potentially therapeutic drugs or treatment and others no treatment at all.

However, in broad principle the distinction between therapeutic and non-therapeutic research is a useful one even if only to emphasise that the ethical safeguards in the latter have to be more stringent. In general the risks taken in medical research are justified on two grounds, first that they may be of benefit to the patient and secondly that they may contribute to the benefit of humanity even if they do not directly benefit the patient. The right of the patient to treatment includes the implicit assumption that they will co-operate in the trial of various procedures but have the right to withdraw if they believe they are suffering harm. The right of the patient to benefit from research on other patients entails that they have a duty to assist in research which may be of benefit to other patients too. This duty is a moral duty, not one which can be forced on anybody. The patient has a right to be properly informed and to give his consent without coercion. He also has a right to be informed of the risks and possible benefits, and to withdraw from the experiment without suffering prejudice in his treatment.

The nurse or doctor in charge of patients in research trials has a special responsibility to protect the interests of the individual patients, to act as their advocate and to advise them about participation and withdrawal from experiments. Because patients in hospital are to some degree captive, it is important to ensure that they feel quite happy about participation in a trial—particularly if it is not one from which they stand to benefit directly. However, staff may also have to persuade patients to co-operate, and here the personal values of clinical medicine and the more universal ones justifying medical research may come into conflict. These may be particularly acute in justifying medical research involving children, prisoners, the mentally disordered or mentally and physically handicapped. In such cases legal and institutional safeguards are particularly important to protect the wider interests of those incompetent to give informed and voluntary consent—even if they stand to benefit or merely contribute to the welfare of others.

The issue of whether it is ethical to use children as subjects of medical research has been hotly debated. On the one hand it has been strongly argued that children cannot be said to give consent that is either informed or voluntary in an adequate sense. Their lack of knowledge and understanding of the implications of medical procedures and even of the legal significance of consent may be said to invalidate any attempt to justify the use of children as research subjects on moral grounds. Their dependency on adults for protection and advice makes them peculiarly vulnerable to moral pressure from adults and makes it doubtful whether their consent could be really free or voluntary. On the other hand it has been argued that this issue cannot be settled by arguments based alone on the *rights* of the individual (child), for medical advances in the treatment of paediatric disorders often cannot be made without research or clinical trials involving children. The right to benefit from new discoveries in medical science carries with it the corresponding moral duty to contribute to the advance of medical research, and this correspondence between rights and duties applies to children as much as anyone else. (Even though we should seek to prevent their vulnerability being exploited where other procedures involving adult or animal subjects would do just as well, or where the risk outweighs the possible benefits.)

Those who seek to justify research involving children (or mentally disordered individuals) sometimes fall back on the consent of the parents or a relative. This can be a way of attempting to safeguard the interests of vulnerable individuals, but the question can be raised too whether the insistence on proxy consent is not more to protect the doctor or institution from legal action. Paul Ramsey has argued strenuously that it is never permissable to use children as research subjects in non-therapeutic research and that proxy consent does not make it ethical either.[8] McCormick has argued on the other hand that since the ultimate justification for medical research is that it contributes to the common good, and justice requires that we are prepared to accept risks ourselves if we wish to benefit from medical discoveries (either in the short-term or the long term), then we ought to be able to understand the principle of this exchange if we have the capacity.[9] He argues that if we do not have the capacity it can be argued by analogy that we would give our consent if we could understand, and further should not be deprived of the right to contribute to the common good merely because we are incompetent to give fully informed and voluntary consent. In fact it can be doubted whether the consent even of normal adult patients can ever be fully informed or completed voluntary, and with children it is just a difference of degree.

In reality, the professional has to exercise discretion about how much to tell, and has to judge whether consent is being given under duress or not. Respect for persons and the duty to care stand in a relationship of tension to one another. A degree of beneficent paternalism is necessary to interpret the needs of the individual, to judge his competence, to decide what is in his best interests. But paternalism can become officious and arrogantly indifferent to individuals if it is not based on respect for persons and their rights. The Ethics Advisory Board of the US Department of Health Education and Welfare has produced several reports on the use of human subjects of biomedical and behavioural research. These have emphasised that three principles are involved in decisions about research involving foetal material, children, prisoners, mental patients and mentally handicapped subjects, namely: respect for persons, justice and beneficence.[10] In any concrete situation the demands of these three principles may conflict and there may not be any ultimately satisfactory conclusion. However if we check the requirements of these principles against one another we are likely to arrive at the best means of protecting the interests of all parties, or the least damaging results for all concerned.

Use of patients as teaching material

Should patients be used as teaching material for the training of doctors and nurses? Should patients with rare or exotic disorders or unusual complications be expected to put up with the additional inconvenience, embarrassment or even discomfort of being examined by hordes of students? In a major teaching centre, where the population do not have the choice of being treated at non-teaching hospitals, should they be given the choice of refusing to act as demonstration material for clinical tutorials, involving for example psychiatric patients or the dying?

Clearly medical and nurse training without the opportunity to work on real patients would be like learning to swim on dry land. Here the justification for compromising the right to privacy of individual patients is that the patient stands to benefit directly (if not on this occasion then in the future) by having trained staff to care for him. Alternatively the common good of all patients is served by having properly trained staff. However, this does not give medical or nursing instructors an unlimited right to do with patients what they like.

The demands of medical and nurse education (like the demands of medical research, health-care planning and public health measures) are such that they tend to give greater importance to considerations of the common good than to the specific needs or interests of individual patients. The nurse on the ward or the junior medical resident with a particular interest in and clinical responsibility for the individual patient may feel very protective towards 'their' patients and critical of the insensitivity of those passing through on a teaching round. This tension between universal and personal values in health-care is well illustrated here. Neither view is exclusively right. Each needs to be tempered by the other. Institutionalised health care imposes some limitations on personal rights, including privacy, but teaching and research institutions and hospitals generally need to be humanised as well.

Justice demands that patients with unusual and 'exotic' disorders should not be given undue exposure to hundreds of students, with or without their consent. Even unconscious patients deserve to have their privacy respected and dignity protected. Lack of respect for the privacy of patients not only may injure the dignity of the patient, but tends to breed insensitivity, callousness and lack of consideration in the trainees. Some patients may be at risk of being over-researched, over-investigated, over-scrutinised because they are 'interesting teaching material'. Some reasonable and just limits have to be set to the demands made on such patients. The duty of patients to contribute to the common good by participating in clinical teaching is not unlimited. Apart from the need to preserve the trust and goodwill of patients by not exploiting them or trying their patience beyond endurance, professionals also have a duty to protect the dignity and privacy of those in their care. This is particularly important if their complaint makes them vulnerable (as in the case of mental illness) or liable to embarrassment (as in the case of pregnancy, disfiguring injury and handicap, or venereal disease).

It may be questioned whether something that places additional stress on anxious and distressed patients (e.g. disturbed psychiatric patients), like exposure to a class of students, is morally justified even with the patient's consent. The tutor may have to decide against using particular patients, however interesting, because of their vulnerability—that is his professional responsibility. On the other hand it needs to be stressed that the expectations of people with regard to their privacy vary according to their situation. People tend to expect the greatest degree of privacy and strictest confidentiality to be observed when they are visited by doctor or nurse in their own homes or see them in a private consultation. However when people enter public institutions they implicitly recognise restrictions on their rights and are often explicitly obliged to surrender some degree of their privacy. (For example, in sharing a public and perhaps mixed ward, wearing hospital pyjamas, in having their medical records accessible to the whole ward team, etc.). In an institutional setting the professionals may be more anxious about privacy and confidentiality than patients are (where much intimate information about patients may be common knowledge on the ward), but nevertheless professionals cannot ignore the need of individuals for privacy and have a primary moral duty to protect the rights of those entrusted to their care.

Allocation of resources

Although we discuss dilemmas of resource allocation in health care more fully in a later chapter, there are some features of these dilemmas which should be discussed here while we are looking at questions where we have to balance the rights of individuals against the interests of third parties. Let us consider a few examples. Should elderly patients be discharged from hospital to make way for more acute cases if there is a doubt that they will be able to cope on their own—even with domiciliary services and support? Should nursing staff be allocated according to need or according to the number of patients? Should more effort be put into nursing those that might show real improvement or should all patients get equal treatment even if their state is chronic? How are decisions to be taken to allocate drugs or medical equipment where these are in short supply?

In real life decisions *have* to be taken and these may be both painful and subsequently found to be mistaken or based on inadequate knowledge. All decisions where the rights or one patient have to be balanced against those of other patients or third parties may involve agonising choices. In formal terms it may be a choice between the demands of personal care for the individual patient and justice for a larger group of patients or society. In practical terms it may be a matter of responding to external pressures and internal guilt and anxiety generated by an unresolvable tension between conflicting duties. The extreme case may be a medical emergency such as an aircrash or train disaster in which many people are injured or dying and there are limited medical supplies and perhaps only one qualified doctor or nurse available. Like similar situations in war time the responsible health professional may have to adopt a policy of *triage*—dividing the victims into three groups: those who must be left to die because they are beyond help, those who can wait for treatment later, and those who must be treated first because they need it most urgently and stand to benefit from it most.

In the case of several patients with chronic renal failure with rather similar pathology and urgent need for the same available dialysis machine, decisions if they cannot be made on clinical grounds would most fairly be made by drawing lots or on a first-come-first-serve basis, as attempts to assess the usefulness/value/importance of individuals would be invidious. Attempts to involve patients in group decisions about the allocation of a dialysis machine would clearly be unfair. In some circumstances, decision by team consensus or by outside assessors might be justified if there were objective grounds on which the choice might be made. However the judgements would tend in practice to be based on the assessment of probabilities on the strength of personal experience or the subjective judgement of professionals. In the case of a real moral dilemma, where there are no practical strategies to avoid the problem of choice, the choice has to be made regardless and the responsible health professional/s have to be prepared to live with the guilt and anxiety which that responsibility entails. (It has been remarked that doctors are paid well to pad their shoulders to carry the burden of responsibility. Perhaps the difficulty experienced by the nurse is that faced with the same clinical responsibility in some situations she does not have the padding!)

In making decisions affecting the lives and well-being of individuals in their care health professionals act as guardians and advocates of the rights of their patients. They have to make decisions based on their knowledge, expertise and available resources. They will have to exercise courageous initiative and be willing to take risks as they try to effect the best compromise between the demands of justice, beneficence and respect for the rights of individual patients.

  Patients' rights and the responsibilities of health professionals have to be considered in the context of the rights of the rest of society—including those who are also patients and members of the rest of the health service. As all of us are potential patients (including doctors and nurses) we have an interest in protecting the rights of all patients. ('There, but for the grace of God, go I.') The right to know, the right to privacy and the right to treatment are all better understood by health professionals who have experienced the impotence and vulnerability of patienthood. The health professional who takes his duties seriously will also be willing to act as an advocate defending the rights and dignity of patients, but will be conscious also that as a public officer he has a responsibility to defend the common good and to promote the health of the whole community and a just distribution of health care for all sections of society.

NOTES AND REFERENCES

1. COHSE 1977 The management of violent or potentially violent patients. Confederation of Health Service Employees, London
  Royal College of Psychiatry 1977 Guidelines for the care and treatment of mentally disturbed offenders. British Journal of Psychiatry, Bulletin April 1977

2. Ross T 1981 Thought control. Nursing Mirror April 23 See also other articles on psychiatric ethics in the same series.
3. Evidence from the Department of Geriatric Medicine and Psychiatric services in Edinburgh does not support the common fear that fire hazards are greater among demented patients living at home. On the contrary, available evidence from the Chief Fire Officer points to most fires being associated with heavy drinking; and in ten years there has not been a single fire among demented patients known to the Royal Edinburgh Hospital and living at home.
4. GNC Scotland 1980 Guidelines on health education. General Nursing Council of Scotland, Edinburgh
5. Fletcher C M 1971 Communication in medicine. Nuffield Provincial Hospitals Trust, London
6. Bennett A E (ed) 1976 Communication between doctors and patients. Nuffield Provincial Hospitals Trust, London, ch 2
7. Duncan A S, Dunstan G R, Welbourn R B 1981 Declaration of Helsinki. In: Dictionary of medical ethics, rev. edn. Darton, Longman and Todd, London, p 105–107
8. Ramsey P 1970 The patient as a person. Yale University Press, New Haven and London
   Ramsey P 1976 The enforcement of morals: non-therapeutic research on children. Hastings Center Report 6 (August): 21–39
   Ramsey P 1977 Children as research subjects: a reply. Hastings Center Report 7 (April): 40–42
9. McCormick R 1974 Proxy consent in the experimental situation. Perspectives in Biology and Medicine 18 (Autumn): 2–20
   McCormick R 1976 Experiments in children: sharing in sociality, Hastings Center Report 6 (December): 41–46
10. US DHEW 1978 Protection of human subjects of biomedical and behavioural research. Federal Register 43 (53) Mar 17. United States Department of Health, Education and Welfare, Washington

6

Nurses and society

Conflicts between the professional duties and political responsibilities of the nurse

In the two previous chapters we have attempted to clarify some of the moral issues which arise in direct nurse/patient encounters without examining the broader issues of the nurse's administrative and public responsibilities. We confined our attention to moral dilemmas in inter-personal relationships between nurses and their patients in order to bring out the nature of patients' *rights* and the professional *duties* of nurses. In so doing we have skirted round the larger issues of social justice in health-care, but were not able to avoid mentioning them altogether. This is because the inter-personal moral questions in nursing arise within a broader social context and the answers we give to questions about patients' rights and the duties of nurses depend on broader principles and beliefs about the role of nurses in society and the nature of the Health Service.

We pointed out in the previous chapters that we cannot discuss the questions of rights and duties without taking into consideration three other principles: *respect for persons*, *beneficence* or the duty to care, and *justice* or the principle of fairness. These are principles of great generality and are very widely accepted as fundamental to morality. While there are great differences of detail and emphasis between the moral codes of different people and societies, philosophers have argued that what virtually all known systems of social morality have in common is their acceptance of these principles. We may even test the moral beliefs of individual people for adequacy by whether they are consistent with these three principles. Recently the Ethics Advisory Board of the US Department of Health, Education and Welfare, in submissions to the US Senate on the ethics of medical research, have argued that these three principles are fundamental to all existing codes of ethics for doctors and nurses.[1]

As we proceed in this chapter to discuss the broader issues of nurses' administrative and public responsibilities and social justice in health care, we will find it helpful to discuss them in terms of these three principles. So, what do we mean by respect for persons, beneficence and justice?

Respect for persons. This principle, while pre-supposed in moral systems for thousands of years, was perhaps given its clearest expression by the eighteenth-century German philosopher Kant, when he said we should never treat other human beings simply as *means*, but always as *ends* in themselves. That is, we should never simply *use* people, whether as research material, instruments of policy or means to gratify our own desires, but should always respect their dignity and value as persons.

While we may have some difficulty reaching universal agreement about which individuals are to be regarded as persons and who are to enjoy the rights of persons, we do nevertheless take it as self-evident that persons, as persons, should be valued and their dignity respected. Respect for persons in this sense means defending their personal rights and, in a medical context, their right to know, to privacy and to treatment. If the moral community is comprised of all those whom we count as persons and to whom we attribute the rights of persons, then societies will vary depending on where they draw the line between persons and non-persons. Traditional Hindu society seeks to expand the moral community to embrace all living things as bearers of spirit. This leads to prohibition of the killing of animals and even insects, and to vegetarian dietary practices. At the other extreme Nazi Germany sought to draw the boundaries of the moral community to tightly that it excluded all non-Aryans, Jews, Blacks, the mentally and physically defective, were deprived of their rights and exterminated. In our society currently there is some uncertainty and public debate about the rights and status of the human foetus before birth, the senile and demented elderly and the severely mentally and physically handicapped, and yet there is a parallel concern for the 'rights' of animals and the prevention of cruelty to them. For example, there is growing concern about the exploitation of animals in research.

Historically, the world-wide reaction to the Nazi atrocities led to the formulation of the United Nations Declaration of Human Rights, but countries like Soviet Russia, South Africa and Saudi Arabia refused to sign it. The world-wide trend, however, has been to attempt to limit the exploitation, torture and killing of human beings by more inclusive definitions of what it means to be a human person. Respect for persons and personal rights rest on definitions of persons, but it has been wisely said that the real test of the humanity of a human society is how it treats the weak, the vulnerable and minority groups. Ultimately we have to make up our own minds whom we will respect as persons.

Justice. The concept of justice has been fundamental to moral and legal debate since the dawn of human history. There are two notions which are involved in justice—the notion of order and the notion of fairness. When Heracleitus the Greek philosopher said in 500 BC that 'Justice (*dike*) rules the universe', he was expressing the view of his contemporaries that justice in human society and justice in individual life are and ought to be the reflection of the lawfulness and order of the universe. Legal definitions of justice tend often to emphasise the importance of preserving social order, while moral definitions tend to emphasise the notion of justice as fairness. However the politico-legal measure 'to preserve law and order' can and do lead to tyranny where justice is divorced from fairness, and justice as fairness will have no meaning unless society has the means to defend and even enforce good order. When philosophers have spoken of justice as a virtue in man they have referred to the right ordering of human life for the good of the individual (and society).

Another way of seeing the principle of justice is to see it as complementary to the principle of respect for persons. If I demand respect for myself as a person and respect for my rights, then I must recognise that I owe the same respect to other persons and must recognise their rights as well. This follows from our concept of a person as the kind of being which can only exist and function in community with other persons. The principle of justice might be described as the principle of reciprocity: do unto others as you would that they should do unto you. Justice as fairness demands that we reciprocate the same respect for persons and their rights that we demand for ourselves. The reciprocal balancing of rights of persons necessitates the ordering of society, and subsidiary moral principles and laws come into being to define and protect that order. Respect for persons and the principle of justice entail one another.

Beneficence. Literally this means to do good. Interpreted so broadly it does not give much idea of what it could mean in terms of moral obligation. In theory everyone is for doing good and avoiding evil, in practice things may be very different!

We have already attempted to define benefience in the previous chapter as the duty to care for others—to do no harm, to seek to preserve life, to protect the weak and to act as an advocate for those who cannot speak for themselves. The Hippocratic Oath (420 BC) gives classic expression to this principle in terms particularly applicable to doctors: 'I will prescribe treatment *for the good of my patients* according to my ability and my judgment and *never to harm* to anyone.' However, the principle has wider application to all men. If we recognise the principle of respect for persons and the principle of justice as fundamental principles each of which is presupposed by the other, then they both practically imply the principle of benefience, for unless we recognise a duty to care, a duty to do something about the well-being of our fellow men, then neither respect for persons nor justice will come about in actual reality.

The doctor or the nurse, in making a commitment to serve in a caring profession, is accepting a very specific duty to care for the health and wellbeing of others. The duty to care is what defines their professions as caring professions, and the willingness of men and women in these professions to make sacrifices to care for and save the lives of other people has given these professions their particular dignity. Because the medical and nursing professions are dealing with people at their most vulnerable and often when they are incapable of making decisions for themselves, they have the responsibility to decide on behalf of their patients what treatment is in their best interests. Making decisions on behalf of children and unconscious or mentally ill patients involves the exercise of what has been called beneficent paternalism. Having the responsibility to decide what is best for other people in such circumstances does not however imply that doctors and nurses are always justified in deciding what is good for other people without consulting them. In fact the duty to care for persons as persons includes the duty to respect their views and judgment. If professionals do not consult patients who are capable of deciding for themselves, then, however well-intentioned their paternalism is, it amounts to an insult to their dignity and may even amount to an assault on their persons.

Withdrawal of labour, or the 'right' of nurses to strike

Strikes and various forms of so-called 'industrial action' have become common place among health-care workers. A variety of forms of industrial action have been taken by hospital porters and ancillary staff and paramedical staff. In 1979 junior hospital doctors went on strike for better pay and working conditions. Nurses so far have been restrained and have not gone on all-out strike, although they have staged demonstrations declaring that they will *not* strike! But would nurses ever be justified in going on strike? What attitude should they adopt to other health service workers who are engaged in industrial disputes involving work-to-rule, selective withdrawal of labour or other strike action?

The Royal College of Nursing (Rcn) Code of Conduct (1977) is fairly unequivocal in its rejection of strike action as a legitimate weapon to be used by nurses.

4. Measures which jeopardise the safety of patients, such as unnecessary treatments, hazardous experimental procedures, and *the withdrawal of professional services during employment disputes, should be actively opposed by the profession as a whole.*

In the discussion these remarks are expanded:

Nurses are entitled to equitable wages and conditions of employment and should be free to enter into appropriate negotiations with their employers. But since seriously ill people are in no position to protect themselves when professional aid is withdrawn, disruption of services by strike action and threats to do so contravene the nurse's commitment to service of patients and should be publicly opposed, whether the action is carried out by nurses or by other professions and occupations involved in health-care.

At the time of the publication of the Rcn Code a group of nursing students commented as follows:

On the subject of industrial action most students think that they have a duty to ensure the safety of patients when colleagues or other health care workers withdraw their labour. A few thought that it might be necessary to withdraw their labour in extreme situations when improvements in standards of care are denied by employing authorities. This action would only be contemplated in extreme situations and only in units when patients' lives would not be at risk, for example in day hospitals.[3]

Other critics have expressed this view more strongly, namely that nurses as public officers charged with the care of patients have a duty to protect and if necessary to take industrial action when the standards of available patient care fall below acceptable levels and endanger the health and safety of patients. This point was made forcefully in the wake of the enquiry into the conditions at the Normansfield Mental Hospital.[4] Here the enquiry found that the appalling standards of patient care were partly attributable to the intolerance and high-handedness of the responsible consultant, but also to the poor state of buildings and equipment, poor staffing levels and poor staff morale. Whether demoralised nurses in such a hospital could have organised effective industrial action may be doubted, but it was argued that considerations of justice demanded that some drastic action should be taken, that in the interests of the long-term safety and wellbeing of the patients the risk short-term inconvenience to patients should have been accepted.

More radial critics have argued that if other industrial workers have the right to strike then nurses, as employees of the single largest industry in Europe, should also have the right to withdraw their labour if negotiations with their employers over pay and working conditions have reached an impasse and there is no other way to achieve a fair pay settlement. These critics have argued that the non-striking posture of nurses lays them open to exploitation by the employing authority—a risk which is particularly great in a huge nationalised industry like the NHS, where decisions about the allocation of resources are taken by faceless bureaucrats or politicians in Whitehall, far removed from the actual working conditions of nurses. Furthermore it is emphasised that it is impossible to separate issues of patient care entirely from the pay and working conditions of health-care staff, for poor staffing levels and poor working conditions affect staff morale and the standards of patient care tend to suffer. The idealism and dedication of nurses makes them vulnerable to moral blackmail in pay negotiations and their compliance only delays the necessary improvements to outmoded services, dilapidated buildings etc.

How do we sort out the moral imperatives in this kind of situation? The Rcn Code gives ultimate priority to the principle of beneficence, or the duty to care, in discussing the nurse's obligations. In a sense this is the easy, most respectable and least controversial line to take. It is in line with the model of the nurse unselfishly sacrificing herself in the service of humanity. However, beneficence alone is insufficient to define our moral duty as it does not take account of the rights of others nor the requirements of justice either to nurses or to their patients.

The principle of respect for persons requires that the nurse recognise the patient's rights, including the right to adequate treatment. Where treatment is below standard to the point of endangering the health or even the life of the patient the nurse has a duty to do something about it which overrides her duty merely to continue to perform her prescribed institutional duties. The patient's right to privacy and respect for his dignity is compromised in overcrowded, poorly staffed hospitals; and the right to know is violated if patients are kept in ignorance of the fact that they could expect a better standard of care. The principle of respect for persons also applies to the nurse herself: she is entitled to a just wage within the limits of available resources and nurses are entitled to defend themselves against being unjustly exploited. What this means in specific situations would have to be examined and the form which protest or strike action took would have to be proportionate to the degree of risk to patients if action was not taken, or to the degree of exploitation or intimidation suffered by nurses.

The principle of justice may also demand that the principle of beneficence be overruled in specific circumstances where patients suffer gross injustice because of inadequate man-power or medical resources which put them at risk, or where health-care staff suffer gross injustice which threatens their wellbeing and standards of patient care. Again the action taken, if it were to be morally justifiable, would have to be proportional to the risk suffered by patients or the injustice suffered by health-care staff. Here it is easy to exaggerate, and the rhetoric of pay negotiations for example (especially when they are conducted before the public media) invariably exag-gerate the 'risks' and 'injustice' involved. It is relatively easy to envisage the kind of extreme situations where strike action would not only be justified, but where it became a moral duty. If, for example, under a Nazi Government a policy decision was taken to perform selective euthanasia on demented elderly patients, one would hope nurses would be prepared to strike rather than implement the policy. Or if nurses were terrorised and threatened with loss of their jobs and banish-ment if they did not do their duty even though paid starvation wages (e.g. under a tyrany or dictatorship) then they would be justified in staging a revolt. However, in less dramatic and extreme circumstances it is is often more difficult to determine whether the nurse's duty to care should take priority or whether nurses should withdraw their labour in pursuance of justice and proper respect for persons.

In the matter of strikes the law in the UK is rather confused. Discussing strikes and the NHS, Gerald Dworkin observes that in terms of Section 5 of the Conspiracy and Protection of Prop-erty Act of 1875 'It is a criminal offence for any health service employee wilfully and maliciously to break a contract where there is a risk to a patient's life or limb.' However he goes on the point out that industrial action within the NHS has in some instances attempted to remain technically within the law by adopting two strategies: a) work-to-rule or work-to-contract, so that the letter if not the spirit of the contract is honoured, and b) by undertaking to deal with 'emergencies' so that those who are at risk are not affected by action taken.[5]

The risk in such strategies is that they become hypocritical. The work-to-contract is in reality a strike with serious implications for many patients—in term terms of unfair delays, deterioration in standards of care or worse if the patient's condition is not life-threatening. The 'emergencies only' policy is a farce when porters or ambulance men decide which cases are emergencies. The difficulty of deciding which cases are genuine emergencies is such such that even doctors cannot in good faith justify a policy of selective action that is designed 'to affect administration rather than clinical care'. As Lord Amulree said in a House of Lords debate: 'The decision to treat emergencies is ...humbug, because one cannot tell what is an emergency.'[6]

It is a common part of the rhetoric of industrial disputes to talk glibly about 'the right to strike'. There is no such right in law where there is risk to the health and safety of other people, and it is even less acceptable that there is such a right in moral terms if it puts others at risk. The fact is that we talk loudly about 'rights' when we wish to draw attention to the injustice we suffer or the felt justice of our cause, but rights cannot be rights if they are exercised at the price of harm to others. Here the considerations of formal justice have to be tempered by respect for persons and the duty to care for others. The alleged 'right to strike' is not enforceable at law but on the contrary often means using extralegal means to bring pressure on employers or the state to yield to wage or other demands. There is a growing concern that, instead of Trade Unions being the victims of a repressive system of legislation which discriminates against them, as Professor Kahn Freund says: 'the danger has shifted. It seems that there is a spreading belief that the law cannot put *any* limits *any* action taken in the course of an industrial dispute'.[7] If any kind of industrial action for whatever cause, however trivial, justifies extralegal action, then there is a serious risk that the law and legal institutions will be brought into disrepute and society be thrown into anarchy. There are those who would argue that such revolutionary action is necessary, because contemporary society is rotten and the NHS in a state of collapse. However the majority of people would not agree and would certainly not consider that such extreme measures are justified to achieve the necessary reform and improvements in society.

However, from a moral point of view, while it may be argued that nurses may be justified in taking strike action if and only if there is serious deterioration of services and risk to the lives of patients, it is more difficult to establish a credible case based on arguments that poor wages for nurses threaten the health of patients. If nurses showed more determination to campaign for better standards of patient care and less preoccupation with their own pay and conditions of work, then their protestations of concern for the welfare of patients might be more credible and their sincerity less questionable.

The moral issue about striking nurses turns to some extent on the status of nurses. If nurses want to be recognised as professionals, and not just regarded as another class of industrial or public utility workers, then they have to act like professionals. The demand for some degree of professional autonomy, respect for nursing knowledge and expertise, recognised status and appropriate financial reward depends upon nurses fulfilling the other criteria which the public expects of caring professionals—objectivity, non-discrimination in the treatment of clients, altruism and dedication to duty, and commitment to care (often over and beyond the call of duty). These values are often incompatible, and are seen to be incompatible, with strategies of industrial action. In a sense nurses have to choose between being professionals and enjoying the ambiguous privileges of that status, including the risk that their selfless devotion to patients will be taken advantage of and exploited, or becoming industrial workers along with all the rest and being subject to the same risks and benefits, rights and sanctions as other public servants or workers.

The difficulty facing both doctors and nurses in a nationalised health service is that it is much more difficult for them to act as autonomous or self-employed professionals might. The greater equality in the distribution of health-care which the NHS was supposed to achieve (and has to some extent achieved)[8] was brought about amongst other things by health professionals sacrificing some of their privileges and autonomy. This was supposed to correct a situation where doctors and other specialists might profiteer on the nation's ill-health.

The industrial relations problems of the Health Service (apart from problems created by the current recession) require urgent attention and in particular there is a need for better negotiation and conciliation services to deal with the pay and working conditions of NHS employees. These changes will only be brought about by pressure from the nursing unions. The unionisation of nursing labour has considerable advantages and gives considerable power to nurses, but it is a power which has to be seen to be used responsibly, within the limits of professional morality, if nurses are to command the respect of society, or society's attention to the justice of their cause.

Dilemmas of resource allocation in health care

Headlines like the following highlight the problems facing health-care staff:

COSTS 'KILLING' KIDNEY CHILDREN
Lack of money and donors deny the young vital treatment.
Andrew Veith reports

'Funds for kidney units are running seriously short. About half the 2200 people whose kidneys fail, die because there are no facilities to save them,' Professor Cyril Chantler of Guy's Hospital said yesterday. 'Most are over 45, but only 61 children under 15 were treated in 1980, while an estimated 90 suffered fatal kidney failure.'

'If there was enough money to treat every kidney failure, we would be treating 1000 more patients a year and would save hundreds of lives. It costs £10 000 a year to keep someone on a kidney machine. A transplant costs £5000 a year for five years. So prevention not only saves lives, it makes economic sense,' said Professor Chantler.

Britain is sixteenth in the European league for kidney treatment. The Swiss do more, and both Spain and Cyprus treat more patients per head of population.

Guardian Friday 15 January 1982

Similarly emotive reports have dramatically highlighted the life-saving character of heart transplant surgery, in spite of the high failure rate and poor survival rate of these costly and still experimental procedures. Dr Peter Draper (Unit for the Study of Health Policy, Guy's Hospital, London) has argued that the money spent on heart transplant surgery would be better spent on health education and prevention, since the heart conditions being treated by transplant surgery are preventable.[9]

Alcohol abuse, smoking, high cholestrol diet and lack of exercise are all known to be contributory causes of ischaemic heart disease, and hundreds of thousands of people are at risk from this preventable but potentially fatal disease. It is argued that expensive 'first aid' measures for a few privileged victims are not justified on either economic or moral grounds when little is done by way of prevention (especially as six out of seven recent recipients of new hearts at Harefield Hospital were heavy smokers and some were continuing to smoke in spite of the known risk).[10]

Two other more controversial examples might be cited as well because they illustrate rather different problems: first, the case of the justifiability of assisting couples otherwise unable to have children to have a child by *in vitro* fertilisation and sub-sequent transplant of the fertilised embryo from 'test tube' to the mother's womb (at present a very expensive proce-dure), and second, the justifiability of giving expensive life-saving surgery and long-term intensive care to seriously de-fective newborns such as mongoloid babies with severe congenital heart defect or spina bifida babies.

These cases may not fall within the area where nurses have much power to influence decision-making, but it is important that they should be discussed for two reasons: first, because they raise general questions of principle which are equally applicable to the resource allocation dilemmas of nurses, and second because issues of resource allocation are matters of general public interest and health policy which are not the exclusive preserve of doctors or any particular class of profes-sional. In fact the judgement of doctors in these matters may very well be questioned because they often have a vested interest in defending the prestige and budgets of their units and related research programmes. Nurses, both as citizens and as professionals with particular knowledge of the inside work-ing of the Health Service and of the practicalities of day-to-day health care, have a particular responsibility to speak out on issues of resource allocation.

In practical terms nurses at ward level have to take daily

decisions about the allocation of resources and are responsible for the use or misuse (and wastage) of costly equipment and resources. Time itself is a resource and the proper or improper deployment of staff has an effect on efficiency and 'productivity'. For example nurses may waste more expensive dressing packs when cheaper wipes like surgi-pads might be used. Or in a coronary care unit nurses may fail to specify what they need and use more expensive and inappropriate intravenous infusion sets when smaller sets with a lower capacity are not only cheaper but safer. More importantly, a ward sister may have to decide how she deploys her staff. In a large ward of elderly stroke patients she may have to decide between giving all patients equal care and attention or concentrating efforts on those patients most likely to benefit.

At a more senior level a District Nursing Officer or Chief Administrative Nursing Officer will be part of the District or Area team with responsibility for deciding on the allocation of manpower, accommodation and financial resources. Nurses have a fundamental responsibility to contribute effectively to the shaping of policy and the determination of priorities on the basis of their unique training, knowledge and experience. Questions arise at this level as to whether or not the management structure in nursing allows senior nurses to represent effectively the concerns of nurses at ward level. In reality doctors may win hands down in any confrontation over resource allocation a) because doctors have the power and the nursing hierarchy is not effectively organised to resist it, and b) because senior nurses tend to be removed from direct patient contact into the higher spheres of administration. If nurses are to fulfill their duties to their patients, to care for them by ensuring that they have equal access to health care according to need and that there is a just distribution of resources, then they must be able to express their convictions about priorities in an effective manner. This may demand stronger and concerted action by nurse managers and staff if the case is not to go by default.

As the examples cited make clear, the issues of resource allocation in health care refer not only to the expenditure of money on life-saving medical or surgical procedures and the use of high-technology equipment such as whole body scanners or kidney dialysis machines. It also refers to expenditure on staff salaries, to the cost of building and equipping new or rebuilding and refurbishing old hospitals, to the cost of medical research, expenditure on drugs, disposable medical supplies and such homely things as furniture, fittings and food. To put the 'expense' of controversial new medical procedures or life-saving medical intervention into perspective it is necessary to give a rough breakdown of NHS expenditure and the proportions spent on these various items. For example, nurses' salaries represent 35% of the NHS budget while home dialysis costs represent £1 million per annum or 2.1% of community health services. The revenue costs of the Hospital Services in Scotland amount to £530 million per annum while a total of £20 million is spent on preventative services (3.8%) and less than £2 million on Health Education (0.4%).'

Some relevant figures for Scotland 1978/79

(Abstracted from Scottish Health Statistics 1979—approximate figures)[12]

Total population 5 100 000   Hospital beds 58 000
Full-time health-care staff 115 000

	£m	percentage of total
Total cost of National Health Service	800	100
Hospital and community health services		
Current	575	72
Capital	47	6
Family Practitioner Services	157	20
Health Board administration	34	4.3
Central administration	3	0.4
Blood transfusion service	6	0.75
Ambulance service	12	1.5
Health education	2	0.25
Research	3	0.4
Hospital services		
Revenue expenditure	530	100
Treatment departments	238	45

Hospital services (cont'd)	£m	percentage of total
Service departments	263	50
Salaries—medical	52	10
nursing	183	35
Catering	41	7.7
Laundry	9	1.6
Power, light & heating	20.5	4
Equipment	13	2.5
Bedding & linen	7	1.3
Postage/telephone	14	2.7
Community health services		
Revenue expenditure	46	100
Child care (schools £10m pre-school £4 m)	14	30
Domiciliary services	27	59
Geriatric	10	21
Midwifery	5	11
Psychiatric	0.8	1.7
Family planning	1.5	3.2
Home dialysis	1.0	2.1
Immunisation	0.4	0.9

The Hospital Services for the whole United Kingdom for 1978/79 amounted to £5.3 billion and the proportions allocated to the various divisions are roughly similar.

However, these facts and figures alone do not enable us to decide on priorities in resource allocation. The duty to care and considerations of justice and the rights of patients are all relevant to the debate and the different weightings we give to these principles influence policy in profound and subtle ways.

Doctors and nurses, trained to deal with the patients who present to them for care and treatment and trained in crisis management, naturally tend to see their first priority as being to save life. Their conditioned reflexes are to give priority to the duty to care—in a response which emphasises their sense of commitment to the individual patient, a clinical rather than epidemiological view of the problem, and a personalist rather than organisational set of values. Faced with dilemmas about the allocation of resources where other patients are at risk, or where administrative decisions have to be taken about the redeployment of resources where the needs of the patient population have changed, they may experience confusion. Where the public are at risk in an epidemic, or where medical research has to be undertaken in the interests of all patients, the duty to care for the individual has to be qualified by consideration of the rights of others and justice in the allocation of resource.

In the first case, when Professor Chantler complains of the risks to children of inadequate resources for the treatment of victims of kidney disease, we see the tension illustrated in his emotive appeal for more resources for life-saving transplant surgery and dialysis machines, while he also admits the need for expenditure on prevention. In a sense he wants to have it both ways—unlimited resources to back up his strong sense of the duty to care for those whose lives are at risk, and further resources for prevention (in justice to the whole population who might become at risk but of whom those affected are only a tiny proportion). Dr Draper's case is based on epidemiological arguments, concerning changes in the pattern of mortality and morbidity in society. Here the control of infectious diseases and effective medical treatment of many life-threatening conditions has left the vast majority of people affected by disorders which are the chronic result of their lifestyle—respiratory disorders and lung cancer caused by smoking, diseases of the circulatory system caused by poor diet, lack of exercise, smoking and alcohol abuse, etc. The argument, based on considerations of justice in the interests of the majority, suggests that priority in the allocation of resources should be given to health education and prevention.

Even if it is conceded that coronary artery disease and kidney disease are in the majoirty of cases preventable this still leaves the dilemmas related to the treatment of defective newborns or the rights of childless couples unanswered. Here, in the case of a spina bifida baby with even a limited hope of survival, the right of the child to treatment and the duty to care by the doctor and nursing staff would seem to override any abstract considerations of justice for others when faced with the concrete case of a child needing emergency treatment and care. The right of infertile couples to medical assistance in seeking to have a child would seem to many people to be a fundamental right. The disappointment and distress of women or couples unable to have the children they desperately want may persuade medical and nursing staff to go to extraordinary lengths, including *in vitro* fertilization, to help them.

However, the paradox is that the helpless defective newborn whose *prima facie* right to treatment may seem so obvious and to whom the staff may be thought to owe a primary duty to care, may de denied life-saving treatment because it is thought to be unjust to burden a family (or society) with a severely-handicapped individual who will make great demands on social resources. In contrast to the helpless infant who is unable to argue his case, forceful articulate and determined couples may be able to exert great pressure on medical and nursing staff to recognise their rights and meet their demands. In both cases difficult decisions may have to be made and these relate to drawing limits to what it is reasonable and just to demand in the light of circumstances.

The objective assessment of the spina bifida baby's prospects for survival and quality of life have to be balanced against what burden of responsibility it is reasonable and practicable to expect the medical and nursing staff, the child's parents and society to carry. Justice demands that these other interests should be consulted and taken into account in seeking an answer to whether expensive life-saving measures should be taken.

In the case of the childless couple there may well have to be limits drawn to what it is fair to expect public health services to provide. Given the low level of risk involved in remaining childless, in spite of the emotional cost, it is hard to give much weight to the patient's 'right' to have a child. Treatment for infertility might even be regarded as a luxury when the main problem is to limit fertility in the interests of population control and the conservation of diminishing global resources. However most medical and nursing staff would concede that couples have a right to assistance, but to what length and at what expense? Justice would seem to demand that such services be given low priority in public health service expenditure, but people should perhaps have a right to pay for such services if they can afford them. Even then would it be reasonable to expect medical and nursing staff to give up time and resources to meet further demands, for example that they be provided specifically with a daughter with particular genetic endow-ment, such as being beautiful, intelligent and musical? Or that they be assisted to choose an indefinite number of copies of themselves?

Discussion of these examples illustrates how in such cases it is necessary to strike a balance between the demands of beneficence, respect for persons and justice.

The nurse as an agent of health and social policy

In discussing the ethics of resource allocation in health care, K.M. Boyd (1979) examines four different approaches to deci-sion-making in this area which he identifies as 1. *ecological and epidemiological*; 2. *clinical*; 3. *administrative*; and 4. *egalitarian*.[13] However these four approaches may be inter-preted more broadly to apply to other areas of decision-making in health care, relating to wider social and political issues as well. As we proceed to discuss the nurse as an agent of health and social policy we will find it useful to bear these categories in mind. We will consider the attitude of nurses and their duty to contribute in a responsible way to public de-bate about the following; the question of how the Health Ser-vice is to be funded, the issue of private medicine either with-in or as an alternative to the Health Service, the priority to be given to health education and prevention, the relative import-ance of high-technology medicine and advanced research in exotic areas of medicine and the need for better primary medical care and community services.

Clinical approach. We have argued in the previous section that doctors and nurses are not primarily trained as adminis-trators, and that this means that they tend to understand their responsibilities primarily in terms of the duty to care rather than in terms of the rights of patients and justice in health care for the whole society. This approach goes hand in hand with a view which emphasises the special knowledge and expertise of health professionals and presumably their right to special authority in decision-making about matters related to health care. The limitations of such an approach are the following: it tends to be very individualistic in its approach to problems which may have complex social origins and consequences; it tends to be crisis-orientated, to emphasise the importance of curative medicine and medical research rather than prevention; it tends to be clinically and morally authoritarian, underplaying the expertise of other professionals and presuming special moral insight denied to others.

Epidemiological approach. Based on a study of the changing pattern of mortality and morbidity in society, the epidemiological approach is more concerned to emphasise the need for objective consideration of health priorities in the light of demonstrable trends and the relative incidence of different disorders. The emphasis on these more objective and universal considerations tends to be based on a concept of rational justice for all, rather than emphasis on respect for the rights of individuals or the duty to care. Given the evidence marshalled by individuals like McKeown,[14] that the major improvements in infant mortality and the control of infectious diseases was brought about more by sanitary measures, public health legislation and improvements in diet and housing than by direct medical intervention, it is argued that less priority should be given to the acute medical services and more to community medicine, health education and prevention. Furthermore, the fact that most mortality and morbidity in contemporary developed countries is lifestyle-related strengthens the argument for primacy to be given to prevention. (The impact of this kind of thinking is seen in *Prevention and Health: Everybody's Business* and the SHAPE Report, where there are strong recommendations that priority should be given to community and preventive medical services and health education. However in the light of the recession the power of entrenched medical interests is shown in the fact that cuts are being made at the expense of these and the caring services rather than the curative.)[15,16]

The limitations of the epidemiological approach are that it is too abstract and impersonal, removed from the emotive reality of individual suffering and the demands of individuals to have their rights respected. It tends to underestimate the visible impact of 'miraculous' cures on the public imagination and the limited impact or credibility of the invisible influence of prevention. It also tends to be too removed from the social realities of poverty, deprivation, ignorance etc which provide the background to ill-health in contemporary society, and tends to underestimate the countervaling irrational forces which strengthen patterns of unhealthy living, including stress and anxiety, economic insecurity and the impact of advertising.

The Administrative approach. The model which preoccupies those who adopt this approach is that of the health services as an industry, as a service industry with a specific kind of contract with health-service consumers to provide health services in return for payment based on fees, taxation or health insurance. The assumption is that in the market for services the client can negotiate his treatment with the health professionals and that health provision can be rationally planned on the basis of supply and demand. The tests of effectiveness of medical procedures will according to this model be based on proper scientific tests—randomised control trials and controlled experimentation. The tests of efficiency will be the relative costs and benefits of alternative procedures, measured in terms of productivity like any other industry—for example by bed turnover or discharge rates. The administrative model gives particular emphasis to a model of organisational and scientific rationality and tends to emphasise the contractual rights of patients and the duties of health professionals based on a business model.

In many respects this is a refreshing change from the beneficient paternalism of the clinical model and the implicitly authoritarian paternalism of the epidemiological model. It emphasises respect for the autonomy of the patient and the objectivity of his rights, but it tends to ignore the fact that the provision of medical and nursing care is not just a commercial transaction like that with any other service industry. The relationship between the contracting parties is inherently unequal and the vulnerability and dependence of the patient demands a quality of trustworthy responsibility on the part of the health professional which is unique, because people's lives and health are at stake.

The egalitarian approach. In line with a more political and radical approach to social justice in health care, this approach emphasises the necessity for changes in the socio-economic structure of society, and active policies of community development and positive discrimination in favour of the socially deprived, if inequalities in health are to be overcome. The Black Report illustrates with a wealth of facts and statistics two basic theses: first, that the nationalisation of the Health Service has brought great benefits to British society in the dramatic improvement of the average level of health of the population and in the more equal distribution of health care and resources; but second, that between the extremes in social class terms the gap has widened in terms of a whole range of health indicators from infant mortality to indices for common causes of mortality that are lifestyle-related. The apparent contradiction between these two theses is explained in terms of the fact that a greater proportion of the population is now in social classes III and IV and less in social class V than in 1947. The general tenor of the report is accordingly that the NHS has been a good thing, that it needs to be improved and that greater resources should be put into areas of serious social deprivation if a real impact is to be made in improving the disparities in health between social classes I and V.[8]

This report was damned with faint praise by Mr Patrick Jenkin, then Minister of Health in the Conservative Government, and most of its recommendations have been ignored, although comparable evidence has not been marshalled in support of the alternative policies, or the view sometimes expressed that the poor have only themselves to blame, alternatively that the fault is in their genes. If the tendency to blame the victim is to be answered then it has to be met by a number of strategies. Appeal to facts and evidence is one. Emphasis on the duty to care and the respect owed to the rights of the poor is another. Appeals to justice, even revolutionary justice, are not enough if they are not motivated by beneficence and respect for persons.

If nurses are to contribute intelligently and effectively to public debate about health and social policy, and it follows from the three principles we have been discussing that they have a duty to contribute to that debate, then the following conditions have to be met: a) they have to be properly informed about the issues b) they have to be properly organised to make their collective and individual voices heard c) they have to be prepared to accept public office and to be represented where these issues are being debated d) they have to be prepared to take both individual and collective action to ensure that justice is done. It is arguable that while nurses wish to be regarded as professionals, that is as public officers who serve patients and are accountable to society for the standard of care they provide, they nevertheless tend to 'avoid getting involved in politics'. All the issues we have mentioned are highly political (with a small 'p'), and nurses cannot afford to be indifferent to these issues because the welfare of their patients, and their own professional standing and job-satisfaction, are at stake.

If nurses follow a narrowly clinical model they may favour private medicine because the quality of care for the few patients they care for in such units may be much better than in the NHS, but the nurse cannot as a responsible health professional be solely concerned about 'her' patients and her income. She must surely in justice and respect for the rights of all patients be concerned about others who cannot afford private medicine, or suffer discrimination because the better-off can afford to 'jump the queue'. If she sincerely believes that the interests of justice and respect for the rights of all patients are better served by private medicine, however, then she has an obligation to produce the evidence and reasons in support of her view. In the absence of such reasons and evidence, that of the Royal Commission on the Health Service and the evidence of great disparities in the standards of health care for rich and poor in countries like the USA must persuade her, against the alleged primacy of her duty to care for 'her' patients or the alleged 'rights' of the rich to buy a better standard of care at the expense of the poor. If it can be demonstrated that the rich can be enabled to enjoy that right without associated prejudice to the standard of care enjoyed by others, and that has yet to be demonstrated, then that might be a practical alternative.

In discussing each of the questions we have posed—regarding funding of the Health Service, private or nationalised health services, prevention or curative medicine, the relative importance of high technology, acute medicine and advanced medical research versus the provision of better primary and community care—perhaps none of the four models taken by itself is adequate. There are elements of insight and import-ance in each of the clinical, epidemiological, administrative and egalitarian models, but each has its limitations as well. Discussed against the background of our three complementary moral principles each has to be qualified. Politics, as Aristotle observed, is the art of the possible; or, as he suggested in another context, it is the attempt to find the best means to achieve good ends in the light both of our principles and practical experience. This means that the pleasure of politics lies in the creativity of finding new and better solutions to old problems, but the burden is also that of knowing that no solution will be ideal and that our principles may have to be compromised to some degree because of the intractibility of reality and human nature.

NOTES AND REFERENCES

1. US DHEW 1978 Protection of human subjects: research involving those institutionalised as mentally infirm, report and recommendations, part III. United States Department of Health, Education and Welfare, Washington
2. Royal college of nursing code of professional conduct 1976. Journal of Medical Ethics 3(3)
3. Journal of Medical Ethics 3(3): 121–122
4. Report of the committee of enquiry into Normansfield hospital 1978 Cmnd 7357. Her Majesty's Stationery Office, London
5. Dworkin G 1977 Strikes and the national health service. Journal of Medical Ethics 3(2): 75–85
6. Journal of Medical Ethics 3(2):79
7. Journal of Medical Ethics 3(2):80
8. DHSS 1980 Inequalities in health: report of a commission of enquiry into the national health service under the chairmanship of Sir Douglas Black. Department of Health and Social Security, London
9. Draper P, Popay J 1980 Medical charities, prevention and the media. British Medical Journal 280:110
10. Sunday Times Magazine October 19 1980
11. Campbell A V 1978 Medicine, health and justice: the problem of priorities. Churchill Livingstone, Edinburgh
12. HMSO 1979 Scottish Health Statistics. Her Majesty's Stationery Office, Edinburgh
13. Boyd K M 1979 The ethics of resource allocation in health care. The University Press, Edinburgh, p 70
14. McKeown T 1976 The role of medicine. Nuffield Provincial Hospitals Trust, London
15. DHSS 1976 Prevention and health: everybody's business. Her Majesty's Stationery Office, London
16. SHHD 1980 Scottish health authorities priorities for the eighties. Her Majesty's Stationery Office, Edinburgh
17. DHSS 1980 Inequalities in Health. Department of Health and Social Security, London

Moral decision-making in theory and in practice

Justifying our moral principles

In the previous chapters we have discussed practical moral dilemmas in nursing in terms of the rights of patients and the duties of professionals, and have discussed the broader social responsibilities of nurses in terms of the principles of respect for persons, beneficence and justice. In doing so we have not questioned the concepts of rights and duty, and have taken for granted that what we have said about respect for persons, beneficence and justice would be commonly understood. In other words we have taken for granted that there is a broad consensus in our society about the meaning of these fundamental moral concepts and principles. However, it must be obvious that we may question the basis of our belief in these concepts and principles. It is also obvious that some individuals within our society do not go along with the general moral consensus, and further, that the form of moral consensus in other societies and cultures may differ from our own. To examine these questions is to become engaged in moral theory and the systematic study of the means we use to justify our moral principles is what we call ethics or moral philosophy.

The aim of this book is practical and therefore we have attempted to keep the amount of moral theory to a minimum.

Most stable societies have a long tradition of law and custom that embodies the established moral consensus of that society. Obviously laws and customs do change and develop with time, and may change very dramatically in times of war or revolution or rapid social change. Public debate (about such issues as abortion, the rights of the mentally disordered, the definition of death, organ transplants, artificial insemination by donor, *in vitro* fertilisation and genetic engineering) is evidence of the way the established moral consensus is challenged by new developments in medical technology. Social changes, such as improvements in the economic and social status of women, earlier sexual development of teenagers, social migration and the impact of other cultures on our own, challenge settled moral attitudes and demand the establishment of a new moral consensus. However, social institutions cannot function without some stability in laws and customs. Some kind of moral consensus is thus necessary for the ordered functioning of society. In a relatively stable society we do not constantly question the moral consensus, and for all practical purposes do take it for granted in day-to-day decision-making.

We do not normally question the basis of the existing moral consensus unless we are faced with a crisis of some sort. This may be a major social crisis or, less dramatically, a personal moral dilemma where we find our personal moral convictions at variance with what we are required to do or where the majority viewpoint differs from our own. Here we are forced back to examine our first principles to consider the kinds of reasons and evidence which we would advance in defence of our moral principles.

Birth, copulation and death are areas which touch on our private lives most intimately and these have traditionally been the areas most carefully hedged about with taboos to protect the rights and vulnerability of individuals. These are also the areas where modern society has challenged the traditional taboos most fundamentally and where modern technology has opened up whole new areas of ambiguity in the traditional moral consensus. Abortion and genetic engineering, fertility control and artifical insemination, euthanasia and suicide, comprise a list of some of the most controversial areas of modern moral debate both in medicine and the wider society.

If we are challenged to say why we think these things are

wrong, or why we think they are morally justifiable, we may adopt one of a number of different strategies. We may say that we just believe it is right or wrong, but do not really know why and would prefer not to discuss it. In so doing we may give expression to the view that moral beliefs are entirely *private and subjective*, that they are based on feeling or intuition and that moral disagreements cannot be settled by argument or appeal to evidence. Alternatively we may argue that moral beliefs are *decided by convention* and that these differ from one society to the next. Different societies arrive at a consensus or some sort of social contract by reasoning together and agreeing to certain rules for their mutual protection and benefit. Other societies may have different kinds of conventions based on similar or different reasons and may or may not recognise the validity of one another's conventions. A third view might claim that there are and must be *objective grounds* for moral beliefs otherwise they cannot be universally applicable and valid. From this point of view the first view leads to arbitrariness and irrationality, the second to relativism. Instead, it is argued, moral principles must be based on the way things are, the laws of moral behaviour must be grounded in the laws governing nature, the laws determining the physical and psychological wellbeing of man.

Moral principles, however we seek to justify them, are important for our day-to-day living and decision-making. They help us to order our moral experience and provide some sort of systematic basis for decision-making. They are both psychologically necessary, to help us make sense of our lives and moral experience, and practically useful, in enabling us to make value judgements in a non-arbitrary manner. In both senses they assist us in our communication with others and the rationalisation of co-operative action. It is because they perform this primitive ordering function of our knowledge and action that we call them principles. It is doubtful whether anyone can do without principles in this sense and continue to function in society.

Agreement about moral principles is obviously highly desirable and makes social life a lot easier and tidier. But how do we arrive at agreement, and what do we mean by agreement? The view that moral principles are entirely private and subjective is hard to maintain, if it means that they are arbitrary and capricious. Such a view would lead to inconsistency in individual practice and to anarchy in society. The fact is that while we may agree not to dispute about matters of taste, we do dispute about moral principles. That is because we recognise that law and social institutions could not function without them and in practice contracting into the moral consensus is a condition of our being able and allowed to participate in society. Underlying our continued and continuing arguments about moral principles is a conviction that moral principles must in some sense be universal and objective if they are to be moral. We continue to seek reasons and evidence in terms of which to establish moral agreement. We could take refuge in irrationality but that is no real defence — either for the sanctity of our own moral beliefs or from the tyranny of those of others. Reasoning together, trying to find rational grounds for moral agreement, is the means by which we seek to arrive at public (objectively acceptable) and universal moral principles.

In whatever way we attempt to defend our moral principles we are bound to use one or other of these three strategies, or some combination of them. The reason why this is the case is that each emphasises an aspect of moral experience which is important in itself. The *The subjectivist* is not traditionally concerned to emphasise the arbitrary and capricious nature of moral judgements so much as to emphasise that we do internalise moral principles, make a personal commitment to them, make them our own and try to live our lives in accordance with them. Moral principles are personal in this sense that they are believed and acted upon by persons, who may feel very strongly about them. This may of course introduce an element of bias or prejudice into their moral judgements and people may not like to have these personal feelings questioned or challenged. To the *conventionalist* the most important thing to emphasise is the public and social character of moral beliefs and their function as necessary conditions for social intercourse and co-operation. He does tend to point out the variations in moral conventions between different societies but not so much to emphasise the relativity of all values so much as the need for tolerance of other people's values. The universality of moral principles can on this view only be established on the basis of negotiated rational agreement and tolerance of diversity. The *objectivist* is concerned to avoid the dangers of irrational subjectivism and a relativism which threatens to undermine the sense of moral obligation, the imperative character of moral principles. He seeks to anchor the concepts of value and obligation in the real world and not in personal feeling or mere social convention. For him moral principles must in some sense correspond to the demands of reality, as he believes the universality of moral principles and their objectivity can only be guaranteed in this way.

In Plato's dialogue *Gorgias*,[1] it is suggested that there are three senses of 'agreement' which are relevant to moral agreement about principles. The first is that there should be agreement between what a man believes and what he does, between what he practises and what he preaches. The second is that there should be agreement between all men that the principles they adopt will be universally binding on them. The third is that there should be agreement between moral principles and reality, between the moral law and the conditions which govern and make possible human life as we know it. These three senses of agreement correspond roughly to the three kinds of justification we have discussed, and perhaps we should recognise that while each emphasises an aspect of moral experience none is adequate by itself to cover the whole complex subject.

Varieties of moral theory

Many different kinds of theory have been put forward in the course of history to justify an existing moral consensus, or to justify particular moral principles. Many have been based on theological premises, others on historical, sociological or psychological theories. In the following summary outline we shall be concerned with some of the most common and enduring philosophical theories, that is, theories that have been primarily concerned to explore different kinds of logical justification for moral principles. The ones we shall discuss are, in historical order, Natural Law theory, agapeistic ethics, intuitionism, utilitarianism and deontological ethics.

a) Natural law theory

In its classical form it is difficult to disentangle this theory from traditional religious beliefs, and this is true both in the

Graeco-Roman and Judeo-Christian traditions. In Sophocles' tragedy *Antigone*, the heroine of that name appeals against the tyranny, the arbitrary edit, of the king which prohibits her from burying her brother. She appeals to the law of God, of universal justice, which governs the universe. The Greek and Roman Stoics argued that the universe is rationally intelligible because it is a cosmos, that is, an ordered whole governed by rational laws. Human reason is just a part of the Divine Reason which is the basis of this rational order in the universe, and that is why human reason can understand that order and should live in accordance with that given order in reality. In both cases the appeal to a moral law written into Nature is, first, to resist the arbitrariness of personal edicts and the relativism of social conventions and second, to explain the universality and interpersonal validity of moral principles.

When the Roman Empire expanded to include numerous other societies and cultures, Roman jurists found it necessary to develop a distinction between the conventional law of the societies they ruled (e.g. the Mosaic law of the Jewish people) and the universal principles of law which they believed were applicable to all societies and by which the justice of conventional laws might be judged. The former was called the *jus gentium*, the latter the *jus naturale*. This *jus naturale* became the basis of what in the tradition of Roman-Dutch Law was called Natural Law. Two traditions developed in Roman-Dutch Law. The first emphasised the Stoic view of the rationality of justice being grounded in the rationality of the order of nature. The second, later, tradition sought to ground the rationality of justice in the rationality of man and the social contracts which he develops to express that rationality.

The Roman Catholic tradition of law and morality has been based traditionally on a doctrine of Natural Law which tends to be reinforced by arguments taken from Revelation. In its classic form, the doctrine is very similar to the Stoic one. It is argued that because God created the world an ordered whole, governed by laws, and man has the intelligence to grasp that fact, he can deduce from the observation of nature what it is necessary for him to do if he is to fulfil his human nature and live a fully human life in society with other men. In theory, that is all that we need presuppose if man is to deduce the laws necessary to avoid living an inhuman or subhuman life, or creating an inhumane society. In practice, the Nature Law is supplemented by appeal to Revelation — to the laws given to Moses and the teachings of Christ. When Catholics condemn contraception or abortion as evil, it is not always clear whether they do so on the basis of Natural Law or Biblical teaching, or a combination of both.

Historically, Natural Law theory in ethics and jurisprudence has had an enormous influence on the development of our social and legal institutions. When Americans seek to test the validity of laws by their consistency with the Constitution (which embodies a declaration of human rights), or when appeal is made to Common Law in England, appeal is being made to principles of justice which are considered more universal than statutory law. The United Nations Declaration of Human Rights, and other modern attempts to formulate universal human rights, make implicit or explicit appeal to the idea of rights as grounded in the nature of man as such, to Natural Law.[2]

b) Agapeistic ethics

This unfamiliar phase comes from the Greek word for 'caring love' and refers to those ethical theories which seek to base moral principles and decision-making ultimately on love. This tradition stems chiefly from the Jewish and Christian religions, but is not confined to them. In contrast to the Natural Law tradition which emphasises the rationality of man above everything else, the Judeo-Christian tradition seeks to define man's essential nature in terms of his capacity to love. In theological terms the argument runs that God is Love and because man is made in the image of God, the most important thing about man, the most important value in human life, is love. In terms of this theory love is not only the ultimate test and justification for our moral principles, but it can also be the basis on which we make specific moral judgements, that is, by deciding what is the most loving thing to do in the circumstances.

Historically agapeistic ethics developed in opposition to legalistic ethics based on religious and ritualistic taboos — whether these were believed to be of divine or human origin. At one level agapeistic ethics is a protest against a conception of God as a God of stern justice insisting on ritual holiness. On the other hand it often takes the form of a protest against universal rules and laws, claiming that we cannot force concrete human situations in their everyday variety and uniqueness to fit the requirements of abstract general laws. Love demands that we recognise the particular character of each unique human situation and the painful complexity of moral choices in real life. To live by love rather than by the demands of laws, it is claimed, is liberating, while living by law is restricting and guilt inducing. Its critics argue that one cannot live without rules, that this anti-law (antinomian) attitude leads to anarchy.

In response to the charge of antinomianism, advocates of agapeistic ethics have adopted two different approaches. The first is to say that there is a logic to our loves which does provide some guidelines as to how we should act. The second more radical alternative is to say that we do not need rules at all, that rules tend to make us prejudge human situations and moral experience, that we must therefore approach each situation as far as possible without preconceptions and allow love to dictate to us what to do.

There are several examples of the first kind. The teachings of St Augustine are perhaps the most famous and historically influential, those of Paul Ramsey perhaps the most important of recent theories. St Augustine argues that because God is Love and man is made in the image of God, then it is his capacity to love which characterises man's nature and it is achieving the right order of priority amongst his loves that constitutes the primary task of the moral life. But how do we know what is the right order? God has created nature as an ordered hierarchy of beings: from the physical elements to plants, insects, animals and man. (St Augustine would add angels at the top of the hierarchy). Corresponding to this order in nature is an order in human life of the physical, emotional, intellectual and spiritual. Man's loves can be ordered in their moral importance accordingly. All other loves must be subordinated to *agape*. Love of God and love of fellow men, friendship, the desire for personal fulfilment, erotic love and basic physical appetite are each important in their own place, but unless each is subordinated to the other in that order then chaos results. Basic physical appetite must be subordinated to and controlled by the others or it leads to selfish, exploitative action at the expense of others and one's own harm. The desire for self-fulfilment has to be subordinated to the demands of friendship and the higher duty to care for the wellbeing of others under God, and so on. Evil is deranged love, giving undue importance to lower loves over higher.

The second alternative, what has recently been called 'situation ethics' can also be traced to a famous saying of St Augustine, 'Love God, and do as you please.' However in its modern form it owes much more to the existentialist philosophers, particularly Jean-Paul Sartre and Albert Camus. Joseph Fletcher, who has attempted to apply this kind of love-ethic to medicine, is of particular interest here. Broadly speaking he is arguing that all that the doctor or nurse needs is his personal commitment to a love ethic and a sensitivity to what each human situation demands. Deciding what is right to do in each case means taking account of the unique circumstances of each patient, the nature of the caring relationship between health-professional and patient and deciding what is the most loving thing to do in the situation.[3]

c) Intuitionism

While Natural Law theories try to safeguard the objective and universal character of moral principles, and agapeistic theories emphasise personal commitment to values and the subjective element in moral judgement, both theories are complex and combine other elements as well. Both theories were historically rooted in belief in a God-made order, although secular forms of both theories have developed later which do not use the God-hypothesis. Elements of convention come into both theories in their practical application.

Perhaps the purest form of subjective theory is intuitionism. It is the theory that we arrive at moral principles by rational introspection, by looking into our own minds and grasping what we find there. 'Intuition' means 'direct perception', 'insight'. In popular terms we know what is right by consulting our consciences. Intuitionism is the view that it is by direct inspection of our own minds that we know what to do.

Intuitionism comes in both simple and sophisticated forms and perhaps there are elements of intuitionism in all ethical theories. For example, how in Natural Law theory one knows which elements of order are relevant to moral experience is a matter of moral insight. Similarly, knowing what is the most loving thing to do in a particular case means considering all the relevant factors and arriving at a judgement by some kind of intuition. At its crudest, intuitionism may represent a refusal to give reasons or evidence for a moral point of view, and a retreat into inarticulate irrationality, but more seriously it is an attempt to draw attention to the activity of the moral subject as an essential factor in moral judgement. Computers cannot make moral judgements; one has to be a human subject, or moral agent, to do so.

Intuitionists have traditionally tried to avoid the charge that moral principles are the products of random, arbitrary and capricious judgement by arguing that there are given structures in the mind or moral experience which we intuit. For Plato, moral principles are in some sense innate. We are born with certain implicit moral ideas which it is the function of reason to make explicit in consciousness. For the early Quakers and certain Reformers, we know moral principles by illumination from the Divine Light or Holy Spirit. In defending the ultimate authority of personal conscience against the authority of the Church they appealed to direct intuition of moral principles. For Kant it is the introspective rational activity whereby we consider the principles which alone make reasoning and the rational life possible, that gives us insight into the form of the Moral Law. Intuition of what he called the *a priori* forms of reason is the ultimate basis on which we justify moral principles.

Intuitionism emphasises two important features of moral experience, first that our consciences are preformed in some way before we come to make moral judgements for ourselves, and second that to be responsible moral agents we must have internalised moral values and made them our own. We may explain the preformed character of conscience as Plato, the Quakers or Kant did, or we may explain it in terms of the process by which we are educated and socialised into the acceptance of a set of values. In practice it is difficult to separate intuitionism from theories which explain the origin of moral principles in social convention. When someone says 'That just isn't cricket', he appeals implicitly to the moral consensus among Englishmen as to what is acceptable behaviour and what is not. The 'intuition' of what is right or good tends to be filled out in practice by content drawn from religious tradition or social convention. However, as we have said, there is an element of personal judgement or intuition in the way we both understand and apply moral principles, and it is important that we recognise this.[4]

d) Teleological or utilitarian theories

Teleological theories (from the Greek word *telos*, meaning goal or purpose) seek to justify moral principles in terms of some overall goal or sense of purpose in nature or human society. Aristotle (320BC), for example, argues that all living things have a built-in tendency to seek and grow towards their fulfilment. As the acorn tends to grow into an oak tree and reproduce itself by cross-fertilisation with other oak trees and so produce further acorns and oak trees, so animals strive towards the fulfilment or perfection of their form and reproduction of their kind. Man, on his view, has a built-in tendency to strive towards his fulfilment as a human being of his physical, emotional and intellectual faculties. The goal which governs this striving is the pursuit of happiness, both in terms of personal wellbeing and fulfilment as well as the happiness of the rest of society, since he argues, man is a political animal and cannot be happy in isolation.

In many respects, this theory has common elements with Natural Law theories, in emphasising that the tendency to strive for happiness is built into our nature as a law of our being, that it is not just a matter of subjective feeling or desire but a characteristic of our given human nature. However, happiness can be interpreted as a psychological state rather than a state of being, and the goal of striving towards happiness can be seen as a chosen rational goal rather than one built into nature. Theories which interpret the pursuit of happiness as a chosen rational goal of human societies have been called *utilitarian*, because the usefulness or value of an action or policy is determined by whether it adds to the sum total of human happiness.

Aristotle's theory has been called utilitarian insofar as his test of the rightness of actions and moral principles is whether they are conducive to greater human happiness. However his theory is more tied to his biology and his physics and his view is that the tendency to strive for happiness is not primarily a matter of choice by individuals or agreed social policy. He would agree that man has to understand and consciously strive for human fulfilment, but he would argue that he is also determined by nature to do so. The Utilitarians are more concerned to emphasise that the goal of happiness for all is a matter of deliberate policy by individuals and society. In fact they tend to suggest, following Hobbes and Rousseau, that the policy of seeking the greatest happiness for the greatest number is based on an implicit social consensus or explicit social contract. In this sense, utilitarian theories tend to emphasise the importance of rational choice and convention. In the work of John Stuart Mill, perhaps the greatest utilitarian philosopher, we find an ambiguity in the discussion of the doctrine. It is that the notion of goal or purpose can be applied to all human activity in a global sense, or to the goal or purpose of specific actions. It is important to distinguish between these two different senses of 'purpose' for the sake of clarity and philosophers have spoken of *rule utilitarianism* and *act utilitarianism* as a result.

Rule utilitarianism describes the view that the utility or value of an action consists in whether it contributes to greater happiness for all. The rule in this case is: 'An action or principle is good if and only if it is conducive to the greatest happiness for the greatest number.' The theory raises two problems. How do we define happiness? By what means do we calculate the greatest happiness?

Act utilitarianism is a more restricted theory that does not invoke a universal rule, but tries to determine in a particular situation, with regard to particular acts, which course of action will bring the most happiness or the least harm and suffering to individuals. It attempts on the basis of past experience to predict what the consequences of alternative courses of action will be in terms of costs and benefits to the individual. It is open to similar objections to rule utilitarianism in that it begs the question 'What is happiness?' It also does not tell us what are to count as 'costs' and benefits' or how we are to measure them. The danger is too that while rule utilitarianism appeals to public agreement as a basis for objective judgements about the nature of happiness, act utilitarianism tends to make happiness very subjective.

Nevertheless, teleological and utilitarian theories emphasise certain important things about moral experience. First, that goals are important in human life — whether they are built into our constitution, or are chosen by us on the basis of social agreement. Second, they emphasise that the practical application of principles and the consequences of actions have to be taken into account in determining whether they are right and good. The element of purposeful choice and the importance of the practical means chosen are things to which these theories draw our attention.[5]

e) Deontological theories

The strongest criticism of teleological and utilitarian theories comes from deontological ethics (from the Greek word *deon*, meaning duty). Kant, the most famous proponent of this theory, argues that it is not the end or consequences of an act which make it right or wrong but the moral *intention* of the agent. It is the good intention, the intention to do one's moral duty, which determines whether an action is morally praiseworthy or not. To get to this view Kant develops an argument about the nature of moral principles which has been of the greatest importance for ethics.

Kant argues that for a moral principle to be binding on me as a duty, for a moral principle to be moral, it must be a) universal b) unconditional and c) imperative. He says we can never arrive at the notion of obligation from an empirical study of the tendencies built into nature, or from the psychological study of man's feelings about pleasure and pain. The concept of duty, he argues, follows as a logical consequence from our notion of rational practice. Human actions cannot be consistently rational unless they obey rules which are universal, unconditional and imperative.

He proceeds to formulate several rules which he calls *unconditioned imperatives.* The first of these is that a man should always act so that the rule on which he bases his action could become a universal moral law. (This has been called the principle of universalisability.) Another of his unconditioned imperatives we have already discussed under the principle of respect for persons, and it states that a man should never treat another person simply as a means, but always as an end in himself. He deduces several others which he claims follow from the concept of duty. There are two main difficulties with this theory. The first is that the rules it generates are entirely formal. They are so abstract and general that they do not help us to decide how to act in any particular situation. The second difficulty is that if all moral rules are universal, unconditional imperatives then there is no way in which we can sensibly decide which rule to obey if we are faced with a conflict of duties (e.g. between telling the truth and protecting someone from a murderer).

Deontological ethics has also developed in two different forms: rule and act deontology. Rule deontology is the view we have just described, and tries to emphasise the objective character of moral principles in terms of the universal, unconditional and imperative character of duties. It is based on claims about the universal structures governing human reason. Act deontology on the other hand is based on a more personal and subjective view of duty, based on intuition, and attempts to determine whether a particular action is right or wrong on the basis of whether a person's intention conforms to what he believes to be his duty. As such, act deontology is a form of intuitionism and does not necessarily make claims about the necessary universalisability of all moral rules. The value of both forms of deontological ethics lies in the emphasis they give to the notion of obligation as a fundamental one in ethics, and to the fact that our ultimate moral principles (as distinct from particular moral rules) must be universal and binding on us all if they are to serve as a basis for both individual and social life.[6]

The role of moral theory in practical decision-making

The range and variety of theories which have been developed to justify moral principles, the most important and abiding of which we have outlined above, may leave one with the impression that there can be no real moral agreement or that it is a matter of indifference which theory one chooses. This would be to misunderstand the kind of impulse which has led to the formulation of these theories.

What they all have in common is a belief that we can and must find rational grounds for our moral principles, that public agreement and objective decision-making in law and the moral life cannot be based on whim and arbitrary judgement. Each of these theories produces powerful arguments for the rationality of moral principles, whether we see the principles of respect for persons, justice and beneficence as being based on natural law, the demands of love, intuition, the requirements for the pursuit and achievement of happiness, or the concept of duty. Each of these theories marshalls certain kinds of evidence taken from moral experience and attempts to generalise its significance for our understanding of the nature of principles. It is tempting to say that each of these theories represents a complementary aspect of moral experience, and that while each has some value, each is limited to the extent that it is generalised as a basis for the interpretation of all or every aspect of human moral life. However there are some irreconcilable aspects of these theories and we cannot rest in such an embracing 'ecumenical' view.

We cannot do without rules or principles to organise our lives and moral experience. Society cannot function without some kind of moral consensus on which to base its social institutions. Law and order ultimately rest on government by consent, even under tyranny. No tyrant can succeed in isolation. He has to be able to persuade others to support his cause. The choice between might and right, between government by force and government by consent, if it is to be a choice has to be based on reasoned argument. If we surrender our faith in reasoned argument, public debate and the possibility of social agreement, then we are lost to the forces of irrationalism, prejudice and anarchy. The only way to arrive at social consensus is by reasoning together—whether it be as a whole society or as a medical care team at ward level.

In practice day-to-day decision making does not involve discussion of this level of moral theory. We operate within the existing social consensus and do not question the basis of fundamental moral principles—unless we are challenged to do so. Perhaps the first time we begin to think critically about our moral beliefs is when we go to school and encounter people with different cultural or religious backgrounds from our own. When we enter training for professional life we are introduced to a complex set of professional and institutional values which may challenge our personal moral beliefs based on family upbringing, education and personal conviction. When we encounter painful conflicts of duty in professional life (for example between the duty to keep secrets and to share information for the benefit of patients, or to choose between the rights of the mother and the father, or to preserve life or to alleviate pain) we are forced to examine the rational basis for our moral beliefs and other people may demand that we justify them. When we move from junior to administrative responsibilities in large institutions we have to find criteria in terms of which to choose between the rules we use for dealing with individuals and the rules applicable to large groups of people. When we move out into public life—representing our colleagues in a union or taking part in local government or national politics—we have to begin to think through the connections between morality and law, ethics and politics. In all these situations, if we think critically and systematically about things, aspects of moral theory become revelant. We do not have to be philosophers to be concerned about these questions. We are drawn to think philosophically if we take seriously the quest for objectivity in ethical and legal debate, and this means adducing the best possible reasons and evidence we can for believing in moral principles at all. The moral theories we have outlined are only a guide to the way some great men have thought about these questions in the past.

Four interrelated factors are involved in practical decision-making: the demands of the situation, the roles of the different actors, the variety of rules applicable and the arbiters to whom we are responsible. Or, more simply: Situation, Roles, Rules and Arbiters. All these have to be taken into account.[7]

The details of a *moral situation* are important. It will involve some general factors common to most human situations and some which are unique to this particular situation. In institutions like hospitals there are general factors common to most patients: their vulnerability and dependency, their need for nursing care and medical treatment, their relative lack of privacy, and in a particular ward maybe the same kinds of medical problems. However each individual has a unique social history, a unique medical history, specific identity and social status, a particular set of family or social obligations. Both general and specific factors in the situation, including those relating to the staff and available resources need to be taken into account.

Roles and *rules* tend to be interconnected. The roles of

patient, doctor, nurse, porter, administrator, relative, all tend to be governed by different specific and traditional rules of permissable and impermissable behaviour as well as general rules governing the institution, more general rules and laws governing society, and universal moral principles in terms of which we attempt to order and make sense of all these other rules. People in a given situation may play more than one role at once. A patient besides being a patient may be a father, a lawyer, a champion bridge-player and a Protestant. The nurse may be a man, qualified SNO, union member and Catholic. The doctor might be a young woman, feminist, keen golfer and atheist. All these factors relating to roles and rules would be relevant in decision making but to different degrees, depending on what was at issue.

When we make moral decisions we also have to consider to whom we are responsible and accountable, in other words who are the *arbiters* of our actions. The nurse would be responsible to the patient and for the patient to some extent (though not responsible for the patient in the same way as the doctor). The nurse would be accountable to her peers, to her superiors, to the doctor and ultimately to the relatives and society. We invariably 'look over our shoulders' to consider who is watching, potentially admiring or criticising our actions. These people to whom collectively we are responsible and accountable, the arbiters of our actions, also have to be taken into account when we decide what to do. While one person might be worried what God will think of his action, another will be bothering about the possibility of legal action against him.

Because all these factors are variable: each situation is different, people play different roles, numerous different rules apply, and we are accountable to a variety of people in different ways, moral decision-making is very complex—particularly in an institutional setting. Having the ability and confidence to make responsible decisions is a matter of knowledge, growth in experience and sophistication, sensitivity and wisdom. While the young nurse may rationalise her disapproval of abortion and euthanasia on the basis of feeling and intuition, the more experienced nurse or doctor may realise that rights issues come into it, and that we cannot ignore the consequences of actions. In fact nurses and doctors 'at the coal-face' will tend to prefer these kinds of justifications for moral principles. Intuitionism, act-utilitarianism and act deontology all are most appealing at this level of relatively direct interactions with patients. Appeal to intuition of what is right (even if it is the echo of the consultant or ward sister's voice) has immediate attractions. Appeal to 'my duty' has the same uncomplicated ring to it. Judging by consequences (act utilitarianism) is particularly flattering to the health professional's sense of his own authority because he is after all the expert in judging what the consequences are likely to be. However when the nurse or doctor has to consider his wider responsibilities to other patients, to the hospital, to the cause of medical research, to society, then rule utilitarianism (seeking the greatest happiness for the greatest number) or Natural Law (as a basis for defining universal human rights) tend to have greater relevance. Rule deontology and agapeistic ethics are perhaps less popular general bases for moral action today, but we cannot ignore the demands of the former that moral rules to be moral must be universal and binding on all, or the insistence of the latter that the spirit rather than the letter of every moral belief is tested by the criterion of caring love.

Reaching ultimate moral agreement may be an unobtainable goal but it is one of the grandest ambitions and most noble ideals of man. If it means agreement in the three senses we discussed earlier: agreement between what we profess and what we do, rational consensus or agreement among men about the principles of social life, and agreement between our principles and the demands of the inherent structures and dynamics of being, then moral agreement is a noble goal indeed. It is a symbol of a fully mature, fully human and genuinely humane society.

NOTES AND REFERENCES

1. Woodhead W D (ed) 1959 Gorgias. In: Plato: Socratic dialogue. Nelson Philosophical Texts
2. Natural Law
      Sophocles 1941 Antigone. Allen and Unwin, London
      Cowen D V 1961 The foundations of freedom. Oxford University Press
      D'Entreves A P 1964 Natural law: an introduction to legal philosophy. Hutchinson University Library, London
      Finnis J M 1980 Natural law and natural rights. Oxford University Press

3. Agapeistic ethics
> Tasker R V (ed), Healey J (tr) St Augustine's City of God, 2 vols. Everyman, Dent, London, Books X–XII
> Fletcher J 1967 Situation ethics. SCM Press
> Ramsey P 1965 Deeds and rules in Christian ethics. Cambridge University Press

4. Intuitionism
> Paton H J 1969 The moral law: Kant's groundwork of the metaphysics of morals. Hutchinson University Library, London
> Moore G E 1962 Principia ethica. Cambridge University Press, ch 1
> Rawls J 1973 Theory of justice. Oxford University Press

5 Teleological or utilitarian ethics
> Thomson J A K (tr) 1976 Aristotle's Nichomacean Ethics. Penguin Classics, Harmondsworth
> Mill J S, Lindsay A D (intro) 1910 Utilitarianism, liberty and representative government. Everyman, Dent, London
> Moore G E 1966 Ethics. Oxford University Press, chs 1 and 2

6 Deontological ethics
> Ross D 1969 Kant's ethical theory. Oxford University Press
> Paton H J 1969 The moral law. Hutchinson University Library, London

7. Emmet D 1966 Rules, roles and relations. Macmillan, London

8. Some general references on ethical theory
> Broad C D 1930 Five types of ethical theory. International Library of Psychology, Routledge, London
> Frankena W K 1973 Ethics. Foundations of Philosophy Series, Prentice Hall, Englewood Cliffs New Jersey
> Toulmin S 1958 The place of reason in ethics. Cambridge University Press